CONNECTION COMPLETE

The *Spiritual* Way
To Escape The Junk Food Jungle
&
Survive Contemporary Stress

A Woman's Guide To Health And Fitness. A Continuum Of Body, Mind And Spirit. Fit, Fun And Free Before & After Giving Birth.

By

Marcia Sheridan, R.N.

CeShore

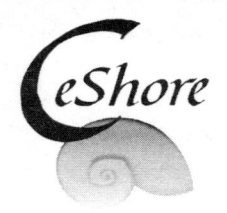

ISBN 1-58501-001-4

Trade Paperback
© Copyright 2000 Marcia Sheridan R.N.
All rights reserved
First Printing—2000
Library of Congress #98-88775

Request for information should be addressed to:

> CeShore Publishing Company
> The Sterling Building
> 440 Friday Road
> Pittsburgh, PA 15209
> www.ceshore.com

CeShore is an imprint of SterlingHouse Publisher, Inc.
Cover design: Michelle Vennare - SterlingHouse Publisher
Photographs taken by - Mark Sheridan
Typesetting: Steve Buckley
This publication includes images from *Corel Draw 8* which are protected by the copyright laws of the U.S., Canada and elsewhere.

All rights reserved. No part of this publication may be reproduced, stored in a retrieval system, or transmitted in any form or by any means—electronic, mechanical, photocopy, recording or any other, except for brief quotations in printed reviews—without prior permission of the publisher.

Printed in Canada

Endorsements

" Marcia came to the American Heart Association with a passion to share her knowledge on risk factors for heart disease and strokes, general cardiovascular health, and stress. She remains eager to reach more people with her health messages. I hope you will join me in supporting her efforts." **Heather Earls R.D., L. Sr. Director of Prevention and Health Care Programs American Heart Association**

" My eyes were really opened"
Vicki Rawling
Program Coordinator
Mundelein Women's League

Food for thought, beyond exercise. Eric and the 50 plus pounds that went with him during pregnancy were the motivating factors for his mother Marcia Sheridan, to get in shape. Are you willing to sacrifice junk food for having a youthful appearance? She began her self improvement with aerobics, and bicycle riding." **Katina Alixander**
Editor of Image Magazine
The Orange County Register

" Marcia, a veteran of the bodybuilding circuit... confident, and entertaining."
Ralph Dehan
Editor/Photographer
Natural physique Magazine

" We appreciate Marcia's enthusiasm on stress relief. It's informative. Marcia's experience in health and nutrition is diverse. Her openness with her personal experiences are to be appreciated."
Felicia L. Yates
Wellness Committee Director
Willis Corroon Corporation of IL.

"If machines don't turn you on, Marcia Sheridan's program will."
David Davis
L. A. Weekly News Paper

"Out of many one people, Jamaica's national motto is clearly at work in Marcia Sheridan."
Music Times Magazine Vol. 2, No. 1

DEDICATION

This book is dedicated to the people who have added life to my life. To my mother, Vyris Preston, a source of spiritual energy. To my son, Eric Sheridan, my hero. To my husband, Mark Sheridan M.D., my purpose for spiritual growth. To my father, Harry Seow, who was instrumental in planting the seed for my life. To Donavan Pigott, my best friend, who supported me since college, but especially for reading my short stories with such interest and awe. To my beloved brother, the late Adolph Thompson (stage name Tony Falcon). To my dear friend, Marguerett Kelly who fought breast cancer to the end.

Acknowledgements:

I would like to thank the following people for their support on this book.

Mark Sheridan M.D. and Eric Sheridan
Bill Unger
Tharone Claybrook
Ian Stevenson
Billy and Ed Lee
David and Walter Wray
Thomas and Joan Hornby
Bob North
Rachel, Sara, and Alice Donahue
Richard Schoeneman General Manager Center Club, Condell Medical Center (Libertyville IL).
Lamb's Farm, Blue Smock and Lake Forest Thrift.
Michelle Burton-Brown (Sen. Executive Editor).
Cynthia Sterling (Publisher)
Mark Kelly (publisher: The Manager's Toolbox, Thresher Press).
Jim Ross (Photographer: Grass Roots Photography).
Annick Rouzier (Acquisitions Editor).
Nurse "W" R.N., Great Lakes Naval Hospital
Dr. Hammond Oral Surgeon, Great Lakes Naval Hospital

TABLE OF CONTENTS
INTRODUCTION

CONNECTION COMPLETE
TAKING CHARGE OF OUR HEALTH
SOME OF MARCIA'S JEWELS

Chapter 1..1
THE PSYCHOLOGICAL TECHNIQUE Of TOTAL HEALTH AND FITNESS HOW TO BE FIT, HAVE FUN, AND BE FREE. TAKING CHARGE OF OUR LIFE'S PURPOSE, AND CONQUERING CONTEMPORARY STRESS.

- Connecting To The Challenge Of Change 2
- How Stress Overload Can Lead To Overeating, Overweight, Poor Coping Responses and Lack Of Satisfaction in Our Lives...2
- The Stress Obesity-Connection 5
- Women Connecting with Women Spiritually 6
- We're Creatures Of Social Learning and Habits.....................7
- Life Is Not Static 9
- Replacing Chemically Polluted Foods In A Jiffy, With A Personal Health Insurance Plan 10
- Body, Mind, and Spirit, A Continuum Of Oneness...................10
- Stay In Harmony With Nature And Our Environment 11
- Humans Are Spiritual Beings With Physical Needs. Nurture Your Spiritual Side..12
- Don't Lie To Yourself, Be A Friend, Affirmative Food For our Spirit...12
- Women As Role Models For Family, Society, And The Future Of Our Planet 13

Chapter 2 ....**15**
HOW TO INJECT SPIRITUAL ENTHUSIASM and DIVINE MOTIVATION INTO OUR HEALTH and FITNESS In ORDER To MANIFEST OUR TRUE PURPOSE.

- Thought Process and Attitude 16
- Breaking Negative Bonds 18
- Confidence Building 19
- Connecting to Universal Energy and Transformation 21
- Self Acceptance and Control Equals Weight Control..............22
- Facing Fear of Failure With Positive Self-Talk and Taking Charge 23
- Solid Goals Are The Path To Our Desires 23
- How To Sow Thought That Will Erase Negativity and Build Our Confidence With Positive Mental Potions............................25
- Don't Worry, Be Healthy 28

Chapter 3 ....**30**
DISPELLING THE MYTHS ABOUT DIET, NUTRITION, SURGICAL PROCEDURES, AND PERMANENT WEIGHT LOSS

- Good Nutrition Can Enrich And Pep-Up Our Lives 31
- Nutrition Control vs. Weight Control 33
- Don't Get Distracted 35
- Taste is Our Servant Not Our Master, Valuing Nutrients Over Taste 35
- What Is Good Nutrition?...36
- Beyond Willpower 37
- Temptations of the Senses 38
- How Good Are Goodies 40
- Making Willpower Work For Us 42
- Eating Disorders 43

Chapter 4 45
OUR NUTRITIONAL UMBILICAL LIFELINE: PROTEIN, FATS, CARBOHYDRATES & VITAMINS.

- Protein Our Life Source 45
- Main Sources Of Protein 46
- Getting Enough Protein as a Vegetarian 47
- The Egg White is a Pristine Protein 47
- Fats: Friend Or Foe 48
- Fat Makes Fat: Saturated And Unsaturated Fats 49
- A Little Lube For Your Tubes 49
- Carbohydrates (CHO), Good, Bad And Ugly 50
- Protein Sparing Carbohydrate Actions.......................50
- Processed Carbohydrates (CHO) 51
- Avoid Sugar and Processed Foods 52
- Simple Carbohydrates (CHO) 52
- Complex Carbohydrates (CHO) 53
- Salt Consumption 54
- The Krebs Cycle 55
- Accentuate The Positive Traits of Food 56

Chapter 5 57
FIBER: THE BACKBONE OF OUR DIET

- The Virtues Of Fiber 57
- What Is Fiber? 59
- Natural Fiber Supplements 60
- Diverticulitis and Discomforts, Stress To The Last Drop........61
- Fiber and Our Hearts..61
- The Human Digestive System and Fiber 61
- Fiber As A Friend 62
- Fresh Fruits And Vegetables 62
- Bran To The Rescue When We Cheat 63

- How To Increase Fiber In Our Diet 64
- Wok Cooking 65
- The Fiber Water Connection 66

Chapter 6 ....**68**
FAD DIETS, DIET PILLS, METABOLISM, AND THE WEIGHT LOSS DILEMMA.

- The Muscle Metabolism-Connection 70
- Side Effects Of A Low Caloric Diet on Our Bodies 71
- Commercial Weight Loss Programs 72
- The Connection Between Women On The Pill,
  Who Smoke 74
- Caffeine 75
- GERD: Gastro-esophageal Reflux Disease 75
- Diet Pills 75
- Beware of Saboteurs, Don't Surrender Leadership To Them;
  Lord Over Your Own Life 76

Chapter 7 ....**78**
PART I
DAILY DIETERY DEVOTIONS TO LAUNCH WOMEN INTO LASTING HEALTH; AWAY FROM OBESITY, HEART DISEASE, AND BREAST CANCER

- Eating Guidelines...79
- Regular Meals 80
- Size vs. Interval 80
- Variety In Our Diet 81
- Avoid Eating Late 81
- The Connection Between Advanced Plans and
  Preparation of Meals 82
- Seek Support 83
- Being Role Models For Ourselves 84

- What's The Connection Between Kids Diet
  and Adult Diet?..85
- How To Escape The Junk Food Jungle of Fast Foods,
  Fast Fat and Snack Attacks...85
- Cut The Grease And The Guilt, Avoid High Fat
  Heavy Hitters 86
- Dining Out Low Fat 87
- Holiday Dining 88
- Why Can't I just Pig Out On Meats For The Holidays?................88
- How Can We Replace Fat? 89

Chapter 7 90
PART II
THE DIRECT CONNECTION BETWEEN WOMEN'S DIET AND THE DISEASES THEY CAUSE: OBESITY, HEART DISEASE, BREAST CANCER, AND OTHER DISEASES IN WOMEN.

- High Cholesterol 91
- Diet And Lifestyle 92
- Lack Of Exercise 92
- Obesity 92
- Diabetes 93
- Dietary and Emotional Stress 94
- The Connection Between Pregnancy and: Diet, Fitness,
  And Our Hearts 94
- The Connection Between Fat and Breast Cancer 95

Chapter 8 96
FITNESS FOR FUN, FREEDOM, AND GREAT HEALTH

- Exercising 97
- Good News About Exercising 98
- Exercising Without Dieting 98
- A Story Is Worth A Thousand Words..................................99

- Check With Your Doctor 101
- Adding Exercise To Your Life 101
- Plan Ahead 101
- Where Do We Begin? 102
- Which Activity Is Best For Us? 102
- Stretching: The Secret To Staying Young Is To Stretch
  And Remain Flexible 103
- Thirteen Advantages Of Exercise 104
- Female Body Types And Responses To Exercise 105
- Genetic Body Types And How They Affect Us 106
- Muscles Can Be Feminine, Savvy, Sexy,
  and Sensational 106
- Pre-Exercise Pep-Talk 108
- Aerobics 108
- Why Will We Burn Fat And Not Muscles? 109

Chapter 9 111
THE SUPER MOM WORK-OUT: GETTING IN TOP SHAPE BEFORE AND AFTER THE BABY

- Before You Move a Muscle 111
- Post-Delivery Isometrics, Toning And Strengthening 112
- Kegel Exercises For Your Pelvic Region 112
- Abdominal Exercises 113
- Abdominal Toning 114
- Pelvic Rock And Roll 114
- Pelvic Rocking On Your Hands and Knees 115
- Leg Exercises 115
- Derriere Toning 116
- Back Rounding and Stretching 117
- Abdominal Oblique Stretching 117
- Waist Twisting 117
- Arms and Chest Toning 118
- Stationary Bicycling 118
- Resistive Rebounding Exercises on the Trampoline 119
- The Mother-Baby Connection Exercises 120

Chapter 10 ....**122**
HOLISTIC HEALTH AND HARMONY UNDERSTANDING THE MIND-BODY CONNECTION FROM A SPIRITUAL POINT OF VIEW

- The Connection Between Sexuality and Overweight in Women 124
- The Connection Between Women And Their Sexuality?............126
- Connecting to our Inner Source of Creation Through Vizualizations and Affirmations 127
- Manifesting Our Feminine, Social, Sexual and Spiritual Self 128
- The Social and Psychological Stigmas of a Woman's Body Image 129
- Affirmations 131
- Affirmations For Health And Happiness for Body, Mind and Spirit 132

Chapter 11 ....**133**
HOW DID I COMPLETELY CONNECT TO TOTAL HEALTH AND HARMONY?

FINDING THE WILL, I WENT FROM BEING AN OVERWEIGHT MOTHER TO BECOMING MISS NATURAL FITNESS AMERICA (BODY- BUILDING).

- How Did I Completely Connect to Total Health and Harmony? 134
- Island Girl Comes To Brooklyn N.Y. 135
- The Pregnancy 137
- Recovering From Pregnancy And Delivery 139
- Breast Feeding And My Weight Loss 140
- Japan: A New Awakening 140
- The Connection Payoff 144
- The Greatest Challenge 149

How to Contact the Author or Publisher...............155

Glossary...157

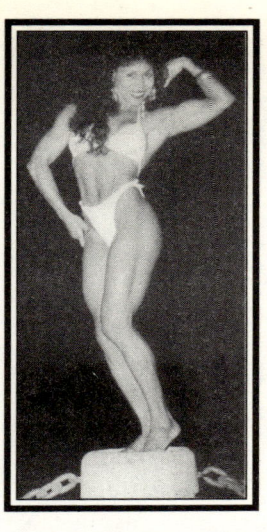

I created a balance between muscularity and femininity for my body image.

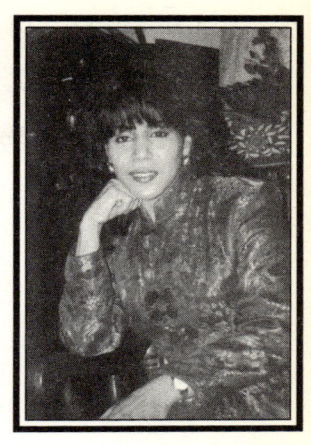

This is me today. No longer on the body-building circut, but still fit, fun, and free.

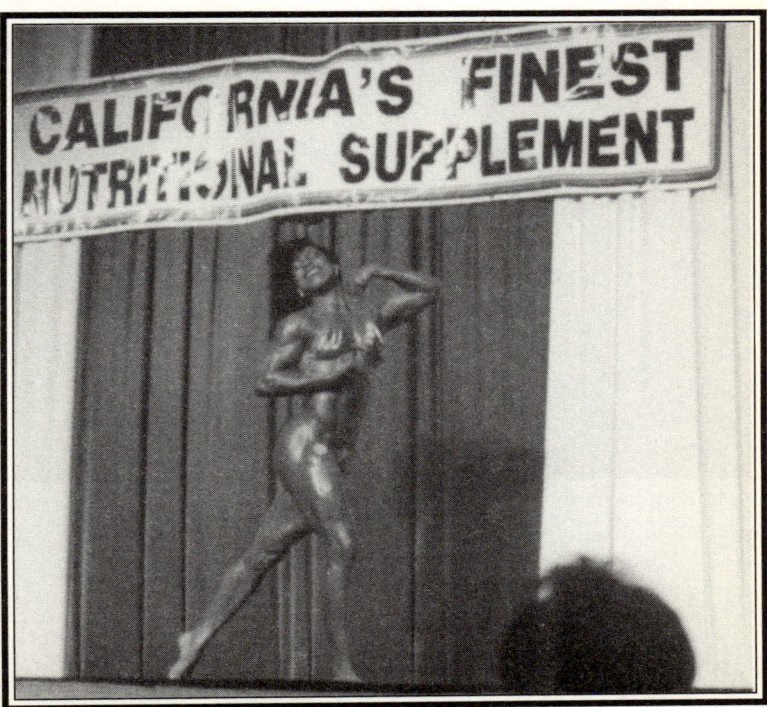

During one of my competitions, I"m wearing my most confident smile.

Barbells from 2.5 to 10 lbs. can be used for endurance strength and toning

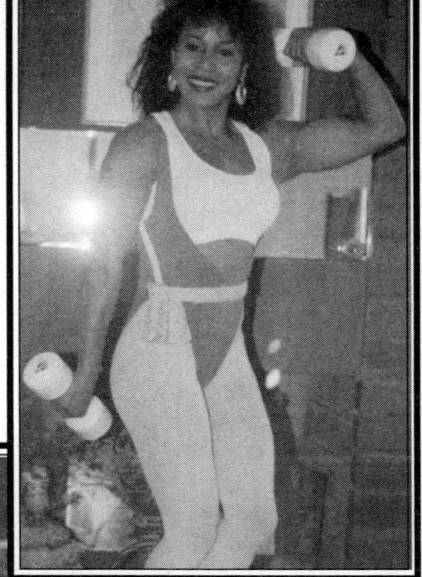

All my hard work paid off when I was chosen Ms. California Natural.

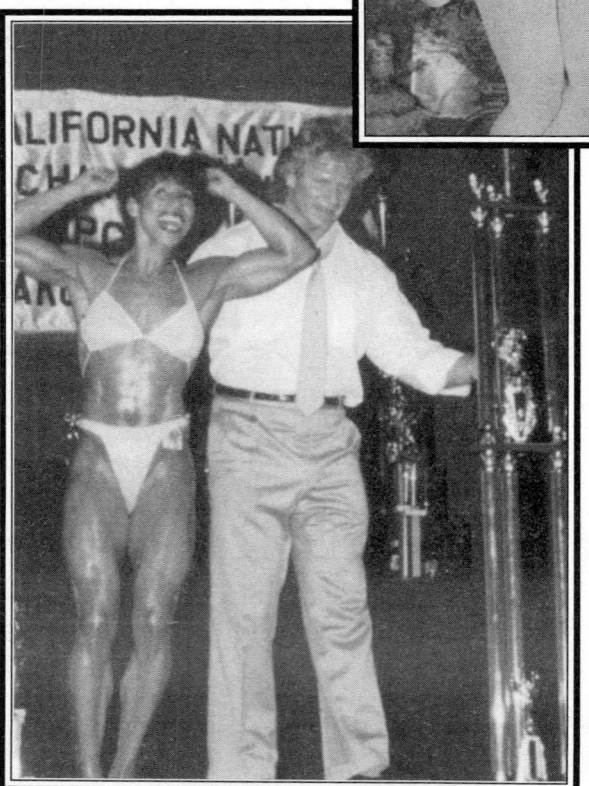

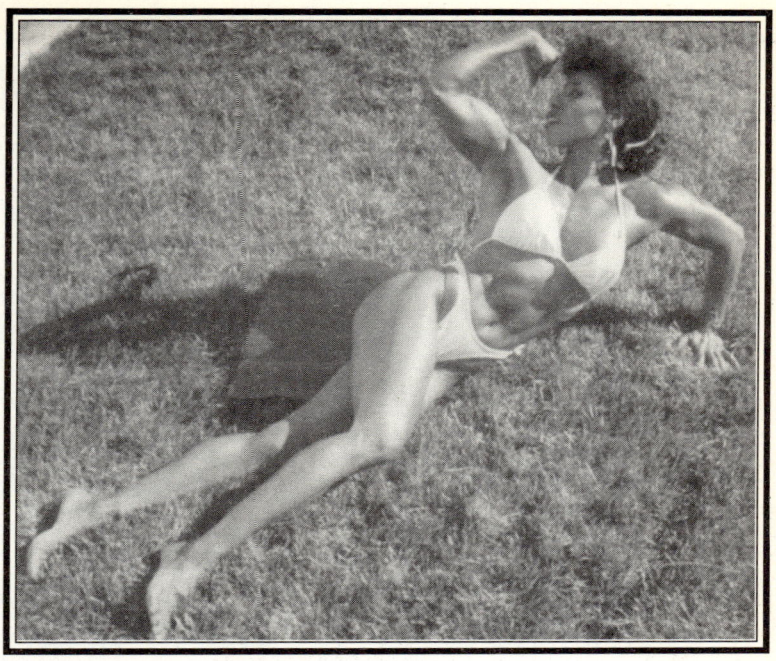

Relaxing in the California sun, I worked on my tan and my body building poses.

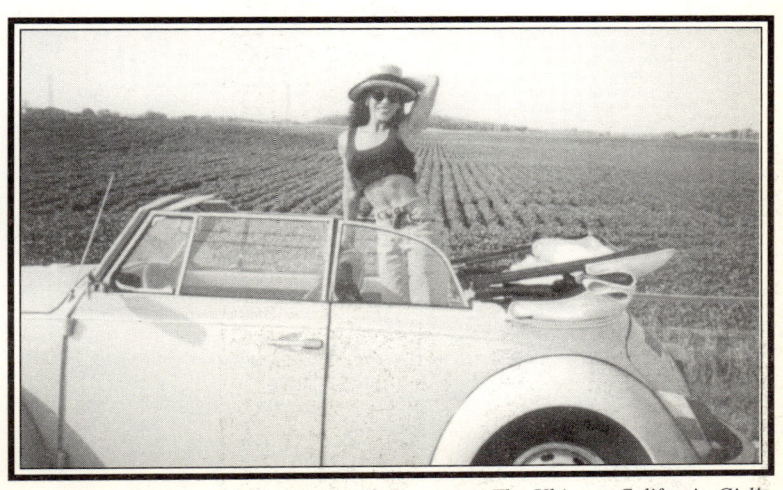

The Ultimate California Girl!

CONNECTION COMPLETE
INTRODUCTION

THE SPIRITUAL WAY TO ESCAPE THE JUNK FOOD JUNGLE, AND SURVIVE CONTEMPORARY STRESS IS TO COMPLETELY CONNECT TO OUR SPIRITUAL SOURCE OF CREATION, OUR LIFE'S PURPOSE AND OUR AUTHENTIC HEART'S DESIRES. WE CAN MEASURE THE DEPT OF OUR DESIRE TO LIVE A HEALTHFUL LIFESTYLE BY HOW WILLING WE ARE TO FIGHT FOR IT. OUR FIGHT IS NOT JUST ABOUT FLESH, BLOOD AND SWEAT; BUT IT'S A SPIRITUAL BATTLE WITHIN EACH INDIVIDUAL. HOWEVER WE'RE LIKE THE INDUVIDUAL COGS CONNECTED TO COLLECTIVE CONSCIOUSNESS. BY CIRCULATING OUR INTENTIONS WE CAN BECOME ONE SPIRITUAL SOURCE OF STRENGTH FUELING THE SAME INTENTION TOWARDS TOTAL HEALTH AND WELLNESS.

This woman's guide to total health and fitness, addresses the complete connection to body, mind, and spirit. In this book, I pour out my heart and soul in a way that will convince any woman to claim her personal power of choice and her authentic purpose on this planet. Connection Complete addresses the growing "Emotional and Spiritual Atrophy" within the hearts of women, as well as the "Muscular Atrophy" without, that leads to "fat hypertrophy". I confront medical issues, preventable health problems, social stress, the confusion of our commonsense and the personal demons we battle daily.

I connect my health and fitness to a delicate balance that resonates from within. I believe that our spirit needs nourishment, love, exercise, and expression as much as our bodies do, in order for us to experience total connection to ourselves and to our universe. My appetite for health and wellness resonates around the quality of life, valuing self and others, non-judgement and compassion for all and universal love. You're invited to meditate, visualize, or pray, to nurture and feed your inner spirit as well as your outer body. Our bodies will respond in kind, in health and wellness to manifest our selves as a whole woman being.

I share with you, a positive, and pro-active fitness program on how to become permanently healthy and happy. This method of complete wholeness has been miraculous in transforming my own wellbeing.

I overcame all odds, not by chance, but by choice. I was just an overweight mother who had the courage to change my life and my future as a woman being. Today I share my knowledge and my desire to serve others through my work as: a registered nurse, professional speaker, speaker for The American Heart Association and The American Cancer Society, fitness consultant, national athlete, author and a woman who went from motherhood to become a Natural Miss All American Fitness champion, (steroid-free bodybuilding champion).

My desire for great health and happiness connected me to a new lifestyle. Connection Complete (CC) enlightens us on what it takes to switch our connection from a culture built on junk food, dieting duels, obsession with food, and addiction to stress to a complete connection to health, harmony and purpose. I believe in being our own auto-body repair person by taking responsibility to prevent unwanted diseases and maladies. We can become a culture of care and compassion for others, as well as self help and the universe will stretch forth its arms to help us.

My old culture is also a source of spiritual strength that helps me to face my weight problem. I come from a culture that values good health and fitness. We celebrate human life, the rights of animals, and we respect the blessings of the earth. Connection Complete invites women to tap into their spiritual force as a unified group, to connect to our ecosystem. We do this by looking within our soul, our intuition and our hearts, individually and collectively.

Maintaining internal and external harmony satisfies our spiritual and mental unrest. It's not just the physical foods we eat that create internal and external crisis. I believe that the thoughts we entertain and the actions we take are the royal road to our present reality. We have the power to exercise a different choice at any point on this journey. We take this step by consciously re-framing our thoughts, our attitude and our actions on the lifestyle we live from this day forward. Our junk food jungle addiction is a reflection of our disconnection from our source of spiritual food. Before we consume junk we first contemplate it. To the degree that we consume junk, we become junk; be it mental, physical, spiritual or emotional. This jungle brings with it the complete circle of agony, stress and dis-ease to our lives. It's like a slowly sinking Titanic ship full of mental, spiritual and physical sleepwalkers. The time has come for us to awaken from our slumber before we sink. Connection Complete is a conscious calling of all women around the world to awaken and exercise our power of choice. A global choice to move in the direction of wellness for all. We can create a critical connection that could move mountains to unite us in spirit. In this state of consciousness we can literally help each other to heal the wounds of our body, mind and soul (BMS). Instead of suffering individually from PMS (premenstrual syndrome) We can collectively connect to our BMS (body/mind/spirit) with the forces of universal spirituality sent forth by each soul. It's a global move whose time has come. Connection Complete is the timely spiritual catalyst to stimulate a global health renaissance of exercise, diet, stress management, emotional healing and spiritual awakening.

Connection Complete is an escape route that is a pleasure to follow. It is paved with personal and professional anecdotes, a sense of personal purpose, and the emotional backbone that women need to change their lifestyle and stay the course for the long haul. Connection Complete informs, persuades and entertains in a unique Jamaican style. It's a fountain of inspiration, rejuvenation, and conscience. Connection Complete believes that self-help, help-others-help themselves, planet-preservation, and global honor, is our only escape to a meaningful life.

Connection Complete brings a galvanizing message to those who need it most. It's diversity comes from my rich multicultural background of Chinese, Jamaican and Scottish descent. I emigrated from Jamaica with nothing to declare, buy only to share my purpose and passion with you. In my last chapter of CC I share with you all about my most personal struggles with diet, exercise, emotional stress, pregnancy and obesity. After having my son, Eric, I was like many women who deal with postpartum depression and anguish about their appearance. I went from climbing trees in the tropical jungles of Jamaica to climbing into the onslaught of the American "junk food jungle". I share how I completed my connection in dealing the junk food jungle contrast. In my native land, some people struggle to get enough to eat, compared to my life in America where most people struggle with the temptation of eating too much.

America is the country we call "the home of the free and the brave". In Connection Complete we will examine the length of our freedom, and the debt of our bravery through the eyes of an immigrant who is just as patriotic as you are. Are we brave enough and free enough to face the fact that we're afraid of pre-mature death and aging. Yet the irony is that our lifestyle includes all the decadence of the junk food jungle, which accelerates our demise body, mind and spirit (BMS). Are we free enough to see that we really live in a culture of full bellies, and empty spirits? Can we see that our spirits are starving much more than our stomachs are? We live in a culture centered on.... fast food, fast fat, snack attacks, and heart attacks. The "Grand Central Station" of supersonic-stress, saturated fat, self-destruction, hungry psyches, and "The American Greed".

America, are we ready to hijack negativity into positively "fit, fun, and faithful truth?". But most of all are we ready to let go of our past conditioning and shape a more spiritual future? Are we ready to stop using our size to disconnect us from others, to destroy intimacy, to inflict pain or guilt on our loved ones, or to prolong our own pain, resentment, guilt, fear, shame, and growth? Leave that jungle behind ladies. Let us unite and become, out of many, one people, with one destiny.

SOME OF MY JEWELS:

All we need to learn about total health and happiness was never taught in kindergarten. Therefore, we must return to the heart of our childhood and relearn the A_B_C's, on how to connect to good living.

It is the underdeveloped child within ourselves who dictates our diet, our thoughts, our pains, and our power as adults; therefore, let us forgive our inner child so that we can re-discover the joy in living, loving, laughing, and learning the ABC's of a healthy wholesome life.

It is time for us to grow up and stop reproducing more of our past mistakes. We are not our past and we are not our mistakes, nor are we a mistake. Weather you're aware of it or not, I need you and you need me. Let's live in the present.

It's time for us women to ask not what the healthcare system can do for us, but what we can do for ourselves, our families, and our planet.

I believe I can be a more effective R.N. by sharing how to prevent rather than to cure preventable health problems such as: obesity, high cholesterol, heart disease, breast cancer and the insults of stress.

It is crazy to expect better results from old bad habits and addiction. Lets plow old ways, and plant new seeds so that we can completely heal our past and hail our future.

We all need a mission statement on our purpose on health. This statement should also be our mantra, which is "We're into health for the long haul."

It is time to experience and express ourselves as physical, mental and spiritual beings. All three parts make up the sum of our whole; they shouldn't be compartmentalized. We must open our hearts to be guided by our spirits, our intuition, and powers of our universe that dwell within us. We must always be mindful that our thoughts are the architect of our world. Let us use them to design the body/mind/spirit that our heart desires.

It is up to us, as women, to calm this global "Operational Diet Storm," one bite at a time. Connection Complete's vision of health can bridge our connection into this new millenium.

Stop cranking cold hard cash into the junk food jungle and unnecessary medical bills. True healing lies deep inside our soul.

I feel that women are the future grass roots globalists to winnow the weeds from our diet and ensure the survival of our children's future. We can be the heroes in our homes, in the supermarkets, and in society. We, too can break old records, and set great new ones.

Let us begin to eat and drink from the bounty of Mother Nature for health, flex our flaccid muscles for fitness, and be guided completely by our spiritual connection. I invite all women to join me: to clean up our hearts and start drinking from the chalice of universal love and sisterhood.

As a registered nurse I am constantly reminded that life is short. There is urgency in my message. This book is an essential tool tailored for women before, during, and after the baby. It gives women a step-by-step, how-to approach to overall wellness. Women need proven tools. They are society's first teachers of the young and caretakers of the old. We are the backbone of society and should therefore unite as one force in this new millenium.

Connection Complete will put a spell on you that will launch your life into the pinnacle of your purpose and your conscious connection to the force of all creation. I embrace you all with ever living, ever loving Jah love, which is one love.

Chapter 1

The Psychological Techniques of Total Health and Fitness

How to be Fit, Have fun, and be Free! Taking charge of our life's purpose, and conquering contemporary stress.

Women of the world unite. Let us escape this junk food jungle and completely connect to our spirits.

The backbone of this book is about complete connection to the different elements of our being. We learn about the natural order of our world, within and without. Connection Complete connects us to wholeness by quickening our awareness on how to be victorious. Here are some of the connections I expect you to enjoy after digesting this book. Healthful foods, fit bodies, peace of mind, personal empowerment, harmony and health, a positive outlook on life, empowering, ways to deal with contemporary stress, making decisions, taking appropriate actions, manifesting your deep desires, transcending fear and anxiety about weight, and getting in shape before, during and after the baby.

You will also know how to connect to your source of energy and courage to overcome the following: stress, feeding frenzies, compulsive eating, obesity, poor diet, lack of exercise, fast-food, fast fat, snack attack and heart attack, poor body image, couch potato syndrome, the fight or flight syndrome, type A personality, emotional burn-out, and spiritual death. Whether you're a teenager, a working woman, or a grandmother, this connection needs to be completed by you.

In this chapter we cover the following:
- Connecting to the Challenge of Change .
- How Stress Overload can lead to over eating, overweight, poor coping responses and lack of satisfaction in our lives .
- The Stress Obesity-Connection in America .
- Women Connecting With Women Spiritually .
- We're Creatures of Social Learning and Habits .
- Life is not static.

- Replace chemically polluted foods in a jiffy .
- A personal health insurance plan .
- Body, Mind, and Spirit, A continuum of oneness.
- A physical, mental and spiritual awakening .
- Stay in harmony with nature and our environment .
- Humans are spiritual beings with physical needs .
- Nurture your spiritual side .
- Don't lie to yourself.
- Be a friend, affirmative food for our soul .
- Women as Role Models for Family, Society and the future of our planet

Connecting To The Challenge Of Change

Because you have begun to read this book, my guess is that you want to connect to your highest self. Congratulations on taking this first step! Maryann V. Troiani said, "Your first step always is to take your first step." You have made a very wise decision to take action now. If we don't now, then when would we? No matter how many times you've tried and failed in the past, you can be triumphant this time. Confucius said, "Our greatest glory is not in never failing, but in rising every time we fail." In my case, failure proved to be my biggest asset. So, together, let's first program and train our minds for continued success by changing our thoughts and intentions. Mark Twain once wrote, "There is nothing training cannot do; nothing is above its reach. It can turn bad morals into good; it can destroy bad principles and recreate good ones. It can lift us into angel-ship."

How Stress Overload Can Lead To Over Eating , Overweight, Poor Coping Responses, and Lack of Satisfaction In Our Lives

Throughout this book we will discuss the demons of stress and it's connection to our emotional, physical, and spiritual wellbeing. Our society is changing at the speed of light, and we're drained and unable to keep up with the demands placed upon us. Some of us overeat, and we eat the wrong foods in an attempt to swallow our stress. Ironically, stress is too colossal for us to swallow, so it consumes us instead. We cannot digest pain without being poisoned by it. Some of us are genuinely ignorant of the harm in the junk food jungle. We attempt to escape stress by indulging in the JFJ. Because of our high stress level, our pain threshold has been lowered, and we're less able to consciously monitor our behavior. We seek pleasure to avoid pain. Ironically, this pleasure is an illusion; it is really suspended pain. Yes, the junk food jungle can fill us with pleasure for a minute, but we spend a lifetime paying for it. Our true craving is for spiritual peace and relaxation. Most of our self-destructive behavior is an attempt to connect to our source of peace and love. We are longing to be filled with love, to be comforted, and cuddled even as adults. But our society has gotten too busy to show such childish emotions. We're expected to dry our invisible tears and keep up with the rat race of life. But, deep inside, we continue to feel empty. We long to be filled. Our desire to find our purpose has us lost in reverie and rapture. We deal with this desire by drowning our stress and our sorrows in a bottle of wine, a bar of chocolate, a pack of cigarettes, or a bucket of ice cream. We lose touch with reality, unable to see that these quick fixes are really causing more physical and emotional stress. We give away our power of choice to the gods of pleasure. Meanwhile, our hearts still yearn for a world of peace, love, and spirituality. We long for the good old days, when people respected and valued human lives. A time when women had more time to pamper themselves, parent their kids, and be philanthropic within their community. We want more time. We want a calmer existence, but stress is where we live. Stress is still our enemy, and the JFJ is our place of refuge. Most of us are too pressured to unwind at the end of the day. Too stressed to enjoy our own company, and too emotionally drained to maintain a positive outlook on our lives. All of this stressful emotional, physical and spiritual exhaustion becomes a vicious cycle. We tell ourselves that some day I'll do this, do that, be this, be that, stop this, stop that, start this, start that, and hama, hama, hama. We're too tired to prepare a proper meal, too busy to eat healthfully, and too lazy to exercise. We drive to a major fast food place for a quick fix. Fast food, fast fat, snack attacks, and immediate gratification is our programmed response to stress. We manage to find the remote control

CONNECTION COMPLETE

as we head for the couch, the only total control we've had all day. We've just juggled the kids around our work schedule, deal with impatient type-A personalities on the highway, beat rush-hour traffic, rush the kids to this activity or that game but don't forget homework. Maybe you're a single mom. The stress is mounting, and we feel like stuffing our faces and going to sleep for a week. We're not designed for corporate stress: deadlines, downsizing, rush- hour traffic, beepers, sleepers, and alarm clocks. How do you spell relief? Have a heart attack. Antacids are not enough. But why do we need a heart attack to pay attention to our true desire and to seek our true purpose in life? Why not do it while we're still at the pinnacle of our personal powers? Isn't our world super saturated with stress? What are we to do? Fight or flight is not a good modern-day option. It was only productive for the cave men. Today there are no hungry animals to kill and no wilderness to run to. Contemporary stress requires thinking skills, mission statements, goal setting, strategic plans, and focused actions. It is for this reason that we need to become aware of the mind-body connection between our cultural stress and our overall health. Our stress is mainly a symptom of how we think. So, what does stress mean to you as an individual? Are you conscious of your stress level? Can you even identify your stress? Do you understand how it ruins our health and wellness? How it drives us deep into the junk food jungle? How do you actually cope with your personal stress? We will explore some of the ways we react to perceived stress. Let's look at four demons that drown us in the deep ocean of stress, namely: Resistance, Resentment, Rejection, and Repression. We journey with these demons, never really understanding their control over our lives. Clients have told me that the reasons they overeat have nothing to do with hunger, but more to do with stress. The first demon to grab us around the neck is resistance.

Resistance is when we resist change, because change is perceived to be stressful. The exact changes we need to make are the ones we choose to ignore. The JFJ is more enticing. It's viewed as pleasure because stress has clouded our judgement and weakened our resistance. After a while, the stress will erode our insides physically, mentally, and spiritually; this is why we turn to our second demon, Resentment.

Resentment is when conflicts are converted into contempt. Our anger is mounting. We clench our fist and we grit our teeth. We're developing steam and we're ready to blow up, but we keep it inside. Instead, we stuff our faces and turn to the next demon to protect us, which is rejection.

Rejection is a climactic reaction to resistance and resentment. In this state we begin to avoid people. We begin to wear multiple masks to cover our fears and feelings, and we intensify our vices. We carry grudges, which can rob us of our sleep, our peace of mind, and our wellness. In marriages, this can lead to divorce and separation. Finally, we become tired of the stress and strain, so we begin to stuff our feelings deep inside to avoid facing them. We then turn to another demon called repression.

Repression is when we claim every thing is great on the outside, but on the inside we're slowly become emotionally paralyzed. We refuse to feel pain, and we walk around faking a smile. We just turn to our sugar and spice and our various vice to anesthetize our emotional agony. Intellectually, we know this is bad for our health, but we need these crutches to make it through the day. We'll tell others that tomorrow we're going on a diet, or we make empty New Year's resolutions. Although we accept food, our favorite vice, we're unwilling to turn to someone to save us from our inner explosions of stress. We develop the hand-to-mouth defense mechanism. As fast as our hands can grab junk, our mouths will open; and, alas, this is how we get trapped inside of the JFJ.

The Stress Obesity-Connection

Forty percent of Americans are obese because they keep their feelings hidden with food. Food becomes a pacifier, solace and love for us; it comforts us in times of stress. Unfortunately, most of us are always stressed out. Do we continue to eat when stressed? No. My goal here is to help us cope with stress appropriately. Because we can't live without stress, we must learn to make stress our friend, our slave, and our savior. Out of stress we can find strength to uncover the best within us. Instead of overweight we can become sprinters with the wind of stress behind us. We begin by accepting what we cannot change. Stress is a part of the fabric of life, a fact we must accept. None of us can survive, thrive, or stay alive without the force, the energy, and the passion of stress. Without stress, life would be lethargic and boring, so let us embrace stress for what it can truly be, energy, excitement, and creativity. With this view we can find the courage to complete our connection and live our true purpose in life. Are you ready to throw this monkey off your back? My question to you is: What bridge will you build to cross over into this 21st century? This book is your bridge. Use it to cross over into good health and fitness. This is not a weight loss book, although we talk about weight loss. More than any of these, this book is an attempt to connect with you completely. It's my choice to share my love and my life with you (the reader). It's based on my own experiences: as a registered nurse and as a woman who was once overweight.

Women Connecting With Women Spiritually

As a registered nurse, I have enjoyed the psychological rewards of both caring for and educating my patients. The majority of these patients were women with diseases directly related to their decadent lifestyle. Although I have taught courses in nutrition to many lay-people and other nurses, I am addressing all women in this book—old, young, thin, fat, career women, and housewives alike. I have worn all of those titles at one time or another. Because I have done this successfully for fifteen years, I believe I can be a positive role model for you; I practice what I preach with a passion. But some of us need to be reminded to love and nurture ourselves because we're so self-sacrificing. We are the educators of the young, and the caretakers of the old, and we form the basic fiber of our society. We need help to maintain our own health and wellbeing. In today's high stress society, women need extra help and reminders in focusing their power. We have contracted the disease called Information Overload Fatigue Syndrome. Women need the knowledge on how to build mental and physical muscles, to balance being empowered with being over powered and overwhelmed. As women we can use our power to help our children and improve our own lives. This book is intended to help you get in touch with the self you love, but haven't loved, as you should. Barbara Deming said, "To resort to power we need not be violent, and to speak to conscience, we need not be meek." The most effective action resorts both to power and engages conscience. Deep in our souls, we know what we must do, let's just take action and do it.

We're Creatures Of Social Learning and Habits

We're creatures of social learning and habits. Humans are one of the few animals who are totally helpless at birth. A colt, a calf, or a kitten can find its way to its mother's milk supply shortly after birth and within only minutes it can walk. A human infant is able only to cry and suck when the food is brought to it. Babies are so dependent on nurturing and social learning they would die if not for their mothers. As women we have power over posterity as well as the present. Let us exercise this power with prayers, prudence, and passion and make our mark now. Whenever I think about creatures of habit, I am reminded of the following anecdote. I met Dr. Joyce Brothers when I was the honored guest of Donna Schuller at the Robert Schuller Crystal Cathedral in Garden Grove, California during the 1989 Women's Conference. Dr. Brothers came over with her breakfast tray in hand and asked, "May I sit with you?" I said, "Sure." We began to chat and acquaint ourselves over breakfast. She later went on to talk about human behavior. She said, "People are not like rats. When you put cheese in a maze, the rats will go down each tunnel until they find the one that has the cheese. When they find it, they stop going through the other tunnels. They only go to the one they have discovered to have the cheese. But human beings are creatures of habit. After they have become accustomed to going a certain way to work, they will not change. Even if there is a shorter and quicker way, they will still go the same habit-formed route. People find it very difficult to change their behavior. They usually have some rationalization for sticking with the same old way". Unfortunately, the old way will not bring new results. Only new actions bring new results. I think it is important to recognize ourselves as social beings and consider what that means. We live in a society where, because we are members of social groups, we are losing control over so many things. We have to pay our parking tickets, pay the rent, and stand in lines. We have no control over the time it takes to get to work in the morning. Rush hour traffic is a stressful part of our world. The news we hear or the news that is available to us sends shock waves that drain our energy. It makes sense to take control over those areas of our lives where we do have some control. We have control over the kinds of food we eat, whether or not we exercise, and what personal habits we must change. We need to take charge while we can. Our lifestyle changes are entirely up to us. We can't just sit back and say, "Some day I will lose weight," or "some day I will exercise." That some day is today! In this society, people seldom die in peace. Life is often prolonged artificially as long as possible, even when the situation is hopeless. At least, we still have some control over our lives. It's time to exercise a little faith in ourselves. Whatever we dream of, we can accomplish. Courage has its own connections. In these days we also need to be mindful that we're bombarded with countless technological seductions. We can become seduced or we can resist the seductions and think for ourselves. TV commercials appeal to the pleasure-seeking weaknesses of their audiences. Little girls are brainwashed about femininity and beauty before they know it. They are encouraged to emulate the toys thrust at them through advertising. Our Psyche is constantly being seduced and manipulated through the media. It is little wonder that watching television often becomes surrendering to our pleasure-seeking nature. Kids are the biggest consumers of the TV commercial junk food jungle. The percentage of overweight kids is at an all-time high; mothers, we must save our children. Even adults are brainwashed into believing that they're imperfect without the right hair color or designer cloths. Overweight women were told that they can't lose weight without weight loss pills. We now know they have had dangerous side effects. Besides most women regain their weight within one to five years after such pills. Women are emotionally, physically, and financially drained by such worthless treatments. We must do what's right for us. We can't allow the seductive media to hijack our freedom of thought. This freedom is open to all of us as we move into a new millenium. Ladies, we need solidarity for the salvation of our planet, and the future of our kids.

Life is Not Static

We're committed to taking our health to higher heights. It's a matter of deciding which of the many available alternatives we want to select. By not choosing to better our health, we are merely becoming victims of the social seduction. Our bodies were not made to live on the processed foods that are available to us today. We need to buy whole, natural foods and eat more grains and more water-packed foods, such as fruits, sprouts, and vegetables. Over eighty percent of our bodies are made up of water. It is wise to keep our diet accordingly. As for exercise, it is vital in providing our cells with oxygen for cleansing and rejuvenation. While our hearts pump blood around our body, it is only when we exercise and breathe deeply that our cells really get some fresh air. Our lymphatic system needs deep breathing in order to rid itself of dead cells and toxins. Oxygen exchange keeps us in top shape. It keeps us youthful and alive; it is what our body needs the most. Just think, it takes only six minutes for us to become brain-dead with lack of oxygen. It is certainly easy to see that our lives can become sluggish when we fail to exercise aerobically. The one thing we need most to survive is in abundance, and it's free. It's called oxygen. We must educate ourselves and our family. What we teach and feed them today makes the difference in their lives tomorrow. It also shapes the future of our society. When we take action, we build our mental and our intellectual muscles. We have to make the choice to avoid putting chemically polluted, processed foods in our bodies. If we put garbage in, then rubbish will be our results. We are already marinating in the juices of our contemporary stress, anger, and hostility. Therefore, we deserve high-octane fuel on our inside to keep our magnificent machinery moving

Replacing Chemically Polluted Foods In A Jiffy With A Personal Health Insurance Plan

Years ago, when we were a nation of small towns, we would go out to the garden and decide whether to bring in some spinach for lunch or some green beans. Healthful foods were our personal health insurance plan. Because it worked then, it can work again. Now, we have to fight not only illicit drugs on every street corner, but foods that act like poison or carcinogens in our body. They are dehydrated, empty calories. Foods that are high in water are also high in nutrients. If we consume those instead we need not drink ten gallons of plain water every day. Ingesting too much plain water in a given day can lead to loss of electrolytes such as potassium and sodium chloride, which are necessary for proper heart function. I think vitamins are necessary in this society of processed foods. Such foods are stripped of their natural properties and their fortification is questionable. Why bother to buy them? There is a lot of controversy over whether or not vitamins are necessary. Not knowing where the vegetables I eat are grown, and not knowing under what soil conditions, I make the conscious choice to supplement my daily intake with vitamins, because I want to make sure my body gets what it needs.

There is a continual clash between scientific and cultural awareness of food. Some familial and social learning of food as love and a socially acceptable avenue for interaction make healthful eating even more challenging. Most of us have learned to socialize around food, to compliment the cook by eating a second helping. To finish what's on our plate. To think about the starving kids in other parts of the world. To break this mindset takes strong conviction, but we can be victorious. When we link food to overweight and pain. Then we can push our plates aside. Then we can say, "no, thank you, I'm so full already," We then are in the process of change.

Marcia Sheridan, R.N.

Body Mind and Spirit, A Continuum of Oneness A Physical, Mental and Spiritual Awakening

When we work on our bodies, our minds and spirits are also helped. Our hearts deal with emotions, and our minds deal with logic. Our emotional sides really want another piece of chocolate cake, but our logical sides tell us no. It is the heart that is attached to the junk food and the old ways. The heart has difficulty working out conflicts because it is emotional. It is much like when you're emotionally attached to some person who is not good for you. It's difficult to recognize and separate from a destructive and dysfunctional attachment. Still, we have to put forth our best effort because we need to complete the connection of our being (BMS). When our hearts are in the right place and we want to lose weight, then we're strong enough to connect to our thoughts and manifest our desires. Just as we can build muscles, we can build cognitive skills. One doesn't need to be skinny or overweight to be healthy. One can be healthy and thin or be healthy and overweight. However, obesity will eventually lead to health problems. Ideally, one should be healthy without excess fat yet not feeling pressured to be overly thin. My philosophy as an athlete is one of harmony and balance between the mind and body. I learned how important this balance is when I was training for body building titles. As the environment, time, and the element change to maintain harmony, a woman can rejuvenate and restore her original shape and beauty. We can all experience a natural balance of good health and stability as within the eye of a hurricane.

Stay in Harmony with Nature and Our Environment

Nature always seeks a harmonious balance. We as individuals can voluntarily rejuvenate and restore our health by making necessary changes that will bring harmony and peace within. Pregnancies and having babies are a part of many women's lives. Pregnancy need not separate us from good health, fitness, and beauty. Pregnancy can be one of life's greatest blessings. I believe the body is to be respected and cared for through regular exercise and healthful nutrition even during pregnancy. The true habitat for humanity begins in the womb.

Humans Are Spiritual Beings With Physical Needs. Nurture Your Spiritual Side

Sometimes we are a little confused about the spirit and its importance. My spirit makes me different. It is the unique inner part of the human being that makes each individual different from everyone else. It is our spiritual side that needs the most attention. When we have external variables like being overweight, poor health, and stress, it is our inner-selves, which suffer most. Our spirits suffer stress deeply even when we're not conscious of it; therefore we must work to unload our daily burdens constructively before we seek solace in the JFJ or succumb to the stress of a heart attack. Our spirits need a daily dose of de-stressing in order to enjoy peace. Meditation is a good way.

I think of my spirit as my guardian angel, and my source of inner strength. In order to have a happy spirit we need to have healthy bodies and minds. A lot of health-related problems, overeating for example, may be symptoms of a neglected spirit. It is the nucleus of our being, and it makes us human. Today, more than ever, people are interested in spirituality and angels. However, true spirituality begins within our own souls.

If we first think of ourselves as spiritual beings, dwelling within our physical form, we will want to feed our spirits with soul food as much as we will want to feed natural whole foods to our bodies and exercise regularly. I believe a healthy body creates a healthy mind. I also believe that we need a healthy body in order to find our spiritual purpose.

Don't Lie To Yourself, Be A Friend, Affirmative Food For Our Spirit

We can refer to affirmation, validation, empathy, concern, and caring as nutrition for the spirit. Just as protein helps build muscles, affirmation is important for the spirit. When people suffer ill health, it is usually accompanied by a void in their spirit. It says, "I have this hole in me, I don't know what it is, nobody cares about it, and I'm in pain." That is why we need to pay attention to our spiritual, mental, and physical being, to see what it is that we really crave. Maybe we need a good friend to listen to us instead of a bucket of ice cream. We need to express love that is trapped inside of us maybe because we don't have kids, or we don't have a husband, or because we do have them and they are driving us crazy. We need to have friendships and fellowship with others to develop freedom to express, explore, and experience the desire of our heart and soul. Friendships and relationships boost our immune system, as well as our self-esteem. They are a great stress reliever. They also enrich our lives and make us live longer. Friendship is sometimes what we hunger and thirst for, more than for the JFJ. Our best friend should be looking at us when we stare in the mirror.

Women As Role Models For Family, Society and The Future of Our Planet

We are women—we're not celebrities; and we're not called heroines, but we all are. We're not professional football or baseball heroes. However, we know that we can be heroic in many ways. Women are important role models for others in this society. Mother Nature selected us as the nurturers, caretakers, nurses, teachers, wives, and mothers. We're the great mothers, to all kids even when we have none of our own. Because we know that all the children of the world are our future. We also drive buses, taxicabs, provide telephone services, work on street crews, serve on city councils, and go to the moon. As women, we are powerful people in action. As role models, we are called on to regenerate, bounce back after the baby, after the divorce, after an illness or operation, and after menopause. We have a second and third adulthood, second and third marriages, and second and third careers. Therefore, we must pro-actively restore order and good health in our lives. Society expects more from us. It holds us to the highest standard of mankind. So let us begin the process of rejuvenation by recognizing our complete potential for power. We try to maintain our self-esteem, handle the grief and the losses in our lives without destroying our health. It is hard being all the things a woman wants and needs to be in a society that seems to be more forgiving of men than of women. Baby boomers are the most challenged group as women. They have had to deal with the most changes in life, yet they're not prepared for the pace. Sometimes our health suffers. We don't eat, or we eat too much, and we become overweight or depressed. How can we fight back? The answer to that question is, emphatically, by rising from the ashes, taking charge, making good decisions about health, and taking appropriate action. We can maintain our health by approaching our self as a whole, instead of compartmentalizing our selves. Our choices and actions should not be influenced by the sexist, hypocritical, social messages. Let's make it clear that women, as people, are okay. However, some of us need to lose some weight, tone our muscles and tighten the heartstrings as well as the purse strings. But we're not talking about losing weight for people to whistle at us. Our heart's desire is to find and practice the fitness-nutrition-religion that will disconnect us from our addictions to junk (BMS). Our authentic dream is truly to be physically fit and emotionally and spiritually healthy. In traveling the path of this dream we completely connect to ourselves and to our universal energy source (love), for the long haul.

Chapter 2

How To Inject Spiritual Enthusiasm and Divine Motivation, into Our Health and Fitness In Order To Manifest Our True Purpose

The new millenium is the beginning of a new milestone in the evolution of our spirituality. A spiritual force that will separate us from chronic physical laziness and diseases, self gratification, mental limitations, and emotional pain. The vertical force of our spiritual energy is our connection to our divine nature of love and physical harmony. This energy fuels our actions making health and fitness an effortless joy. It is time to re-connect to the spiritual enthusiasm that is already available to us. The magic of our lives is the work we put into it. Our success comes in **I CANS**, not in **I CANNOTS, in the spirit we can do all things.** *When we keep the flames of desire and motivation burning in our hearts and minds, our spirit intervene and we're able to move mountains.* The old saying is "great things happen when men and mountains meet." We need to focus our thoughts and energy on the right path for our individual needs. But first we must choose an authentic lifestyle over just losing weight. In keeping our minds focused on our actions we will move forward harmoniously. Diligent thoughts and actions taken in small steps are a sure way to connect to our divine purpose.

In this chapter, we will explore the following:
- Thought Process and Attitude .
- Breaking Negative Bonds .
- Confidence Building .
- Connecting To Universal Energy and Transformation .
- Self Acceptance and Self Control Equals Weight Control.
- Facing Fear of Failure With Positive Self Talk And Taking Charge •Solid Goals Are The Path To Our Desires .
- How To Sow Thoughts That Will Erase Negativity and Build Our Confidence With Positive Mental Potions.
- Don't Worry, Be Healthy.

CONNECTION COMPLETE

Thought Process and Attitude

In order to debunk some of our destructive desires towards food, we need to, **KNOW WHERE OUR THOUGHTS ARE AT ALL TIMES**. In doing so, we can manifest the miracle of mindfulness, self-control, and the power of our own spirituality. keeping in mind that our battle with weight control is physical, yes, but even more it's a mental and spiritual battle played out through the weakness of our humanity. Because we are created as spirit and mind within a mortal body we can achieve our weight control and fitness by tapping into our internal source of power. This is our divine way of getting something for nothing. All we need to do is to ask, expecting to receive, and we will. We need not continue to fixate on our external weight, or the limitation of our five senses when we can internally connect to our intuition. This is a direct way to receive our spirit's instructions on how to achieve our heart's desire. Let's face it, we know that our overweight is mostly a manifestation of our internal overweight overflowing to our outside.

Therefore it's only wise to begin the weight loss from within. A simple beginning is to ask ourselves provocative questions that can awaken, enlighten, and empower us to change our destructive thoughts, behavior, and lifestyle and connect to the path of a purposeful and wholesome lifestyle. We can find divine answers in our own magnificent minds and spirit. Because the answers are partially built into our authentic questions. For example, instead of continually asking ourselves negative questions such as, "Why can't I ever lose weight permanently," a better question is "What is the most healthful way for me to lose my weight and keep it off?"

Avoid asking negative questions with words like never. Our spirit doesn't respond to negativity. Such questions grieves our spirit and drain its energy and cause us additional emotional stress. Becoming over stressed in this way is the complete opposite of being spirit filled, energized and completely connected to our internal source of power. We can turn our frustration, fear, anxiety, stress and pain of being overweight around, by breaking destructive unhealthy patterns. We don't have to succumb to social seductions. We can take charge of our own affairs with the connections we make. On one hand connection can be powerful and on the other hand disconnection can be using our spirit's wisdom. My fear of remaining fat and becoming unhappy was the catalyst that connected me to my inner source. But in order to do so, I had to consciously disconnect from my fear of failure, my fear of poor health and fitness, and my lack of confidence. When we say, **"I want"** on one hand, and yet on the other hand, say, **"I can't,"** we are in fact actually making the statement of **"I CAN'T WANT."** This train of thought further re-enforces our self-doubt and weakens our confidence. We must believe we can do what we desire and be what we want to be in order to enjoy the fruits of our spirit. In order to spiritually to receive our attract our heart's divine desire. We can never "choose" to not want, to want is to be alive and to be human. We can all reverse our childhood conditioning by reprogramming ourselves to do what's right for us. For example, when we have a craving for an ice-cream cone, we can start to develop a good adult habit by grabbing an apple instead. Grabbing a healthful snacks in place of junk food gives us leverage to resist garbage; it also gives us an anchor against such temptation. It will feel strange at first, but keep at it. As babies, it was frustrating to fall but we kept trying until we could walk. Through such positive actions, we can break out of self-destructive chains and connect to healthy living. Don't think about anything else but your purpose; you want to get healthy, so just eat healthfully. In time you'll love it. Once we successfully reprogram our thought patterns with a desire to eat healthier diets, our behavior will gradually become effortless. To speed up this process and really drive it home, we must link the momentary pleasure of the junk food jungle to the permanent pain that it brings. We should always remind ourselves, that this is not what we desire for our lives; indeed, our purpose is to be healthy, and happy. We must practice kizan the Japanese word for never ending improvement. We need to persevere until it sinks into our unconscious that our craving for junk foods and our lack of exercise will bring great pain, unwanted pounds, lethargy, premature aging, diseases, and a poor quality of life. These are all very real end results that we cannot afford to overlook. In contrast, we must also link the pleasure we will enjoy when we touch the apple, smell the apple, bite the apple, and taste the apple juice. Imagine the joy we'll feel when we begin to lose weight, and look great. We must do this for ourselves because we're worth it. We cannot in good conscience give our life and our divine purpose away like a nickel in a slot machine. We are worth the effort and the time. After all we spend more money and more time manicuring our nails. Don't worry be healthy. This is not the Garden of Eden an apple a day is OK. And if that's the first little step you're ready to take I applaud you. In fact, I encourage you to eventually make all fruits a staple in your diet from now on. According to current research, it takes some of us up to six months to acquire a new habit, so it's wise to begin that new healthy habit today. Remember, every time we crave something unhealthy and laden with fat and calories (e.g., burgers, fries, and milk-shakes), and we indulge our cravings, we in fact, reinforce the bad habit, telling ourselves we can't do it. We make food our master instead of our servant. Don't worry, be healthy because we can turn these cravings into small stepping stones to consciously challenge ourselves. In the meantime also consciously reinforcing healthful habits one bite at a time, one day at a time. The magic of change lies in our consistent counter-action with new positive behaviors. WE MUST CONNECT our POWER to our Commitments, so that what we say matches what we do at all times. This is how we purposefully inject spiritual enthusiasm into our souls to bring about positive permanent change. We have no substitute for a positive action. Don't say, "I'll try." Say, "I did", because I wanted to" — and I did it with conviction! Universal spirit responds to our faith when it's in positive action; It's called faith in action. Some of us need to search our hearts for clarity in order to bring about lasting healthy changes. We know that our spirits can best woo us, and guide us through the sea of destruction, the JFJ, and our contemporary stress. Remember our mantra. We're in this for the long haul, so let us continue to seek strength from our spiritual source.

Breaking Negative Bonds

Breaking negative behavior patterns will gradually bring us positive results. These results help us to stop doubting our ability to change. We may have forgotten what good eating is all about, but we've just positively jumped back on the right track by being pro-active. Our first step is the start of a billion miles. That first, simple step of faith will make the difference. When we allow ourselves to be successful with one thing, we will become the masters of many things. We can begin by ruling over our own diet. After we make it through our first meal okay, we can continue to take one meal at a time. I do not believe in putting people on weight loss diets. **DIET** can be a dirty, four-letter word that spells death in the first three letters alone. **DIE...T.** Let us break this negative bond of death from our lives. When I use the word diet, I'm simply referring to our meals, I believe that putting anyone on a prescribed, regimented diet is a big, fat, negative step because it sets us up to fail. Most people are not able to stick to rigid diets for very long. We become bored, our bodies rebel, we get angry and we feel deprived over time. A rigid diet only serves to re-enforce negative behavior. It does not lends itself to a lasting healthy lifestyle. The key to breaking negative bonds is to keep clear in our minds the pain of the old way. The purpose of this pain is to help us to choose wisely in the future.

Confidence Building

Confidence is best built with our minds. Confidence is built through one's own action. It cannot be bought or collected from others. However, it can be conveyed and stimulated by others to be manifested by us. If someone else planned all our meals, we would be denied the chance for hands on, do-it-ourselves practice of using our own knowledge, power, and creativity. Personal involvement is a must; it's the only way we can learn and do for ourselves. I am advocating self-help here, because I believe that if we're willing to help ourselves, we'll get the best help possible, if we just take action. A child has to walk for himself or herself. No one can do it for him/her. That's how kids build confidence, and so it is for us adults. To give our powers away can render ourselves totally helpless. It decreases our mental involvement, and definitely limits our full commitment and responsibility to discriminate intelligently

CONNECTION COMPLETE

by using our knowledge of nutrition. In reading this book you will learn all this and be able to live it for a lifetime. Building our knowledge of nutrition and exercise is the best way to reinforce good healthy habits. Never give away personal power—always build on it and become stronger. We all possess the power to transform ourselves at any time. My purpose in writing this book is to inform and to educate people. It is certainly not to turn them into slaves of my recipes and diet plans. My only intention is to remind and reinforce the message to women that we already have the power within us to change. I hope to help you to find your own empowerment and to galvanize you into action- NOW! Realistically, it is only in the Now that we can change our future. All I have are the words in this book. Words that I hope will move you into a healthier lifestyle.

Words are powerful when we put them into action. Personally, I have never been on a diet program. What I did was to educate myself about nutrition and avoid eating foods that were hazardous to my health. I also developed a regular exercise program to keep my metabolism high. I have remained committed to this lifestyle for the past fifteen years. While most people regain their original weight along with several extra pounds faster than the sun can set.

I have not gained an ounce. In fact, I am still losing fat and toning muscles. As I get older I get leaner; this is a direct result of my low-fat diet. Over the years my body has grown accustomed to less fat and is now unable to digest a lot of fat. I know this because when I do I get sick Therefore, I have lost the urge to eat fatty foods. I've discovered that the secret of staying lean is to cut back on fat long enough to the point where our bodies no longer have the capacity to digest a lot of it. With discipline and commitment, I was able to discover this pearl for myself. Now it's yours too, I'm very pleased. I have learned that by sticking to my goals I can reap greater rewards than I could have expected. Such persistent behavior produces results and builds confidence. You, too, can discover this truth for yourself and stop lusting after leanness, but indeed, be a lean, clean productive machine. Together we can prevent diseases.

I'm not acting as your nurse, but rather as your coach. Connecting with you through this book is my way of completing my connection with you and with our universal source of love. In sharing this book with you I feel far more connected to you than if I were to meet you in a hospital bed. I believe preventing diseases is much more rewarding than curing them. NOW is when I can help you to prevent health problems and to enjoy good health.

I want you to look like you . . . beautiful. My Taking Charge Weight Stabilization System is very simple. It's a process by which one will permanently maintain good health and fitness. It's about controlling weight through proper, healthful eating and a variety of different forms of exercises. It is about making decisions and taking action. It's about commitment and responsibility to our own physical and mental well being, and it's about redemption. We can begin by, first, learning how to be our own best friend. We can teach ourselves how to lose weight just as we can teach ourselves how to fish. There are a few things that only we can do for ourselves; no one can lose weight for us. No commitment made by others can be as effective and powerful as the commitments we make ourselves. So please let it be your own burning desire and choice to follow the path of change. Weight-loss and stabilization can be challenging, but this is what we want, and what we need; a healthy body, mind, and spirit. Notice how often we can change our mind in one minute? Can we totally change our bodies that fast? No, we can't. But why not use the speed, and power of our minds to speed up the change of our bodies? Let the buzz begin, start flapping your wings; change is always in our favor, whenever it's deeply desired.

Connecting To Universal Energy And Transformation.

We'll soon go through a metamorphosis, the way a caterpillar transforms into a butterfly. We can freely fly out of the JFJ jungle, by transcending beyond our physical form and our five senses. We do this by internalizing towards our intuition, which is the conscious connection to our spirit. This is how we can put our positive intentions for health and happiness into the universe. We send this energy out for ourselves and to each other just by our intention. We must first give away what ever we would like for our own prosperity. The African proverb says, "Health of the body is prosperity." As an individual or as a group, we can enjoy this prosperity simply by sending our intent. I believe our life's course is always a manifestation of our current intent or desire. As we give with open hearts we will receive spiritual love and energy from others. Each of us has a spiritual gift for the healing of our collective body. Until we all become clear that we're interconnected and dependent on each other's gift we will not enjoy true healing of our BMS as a unified spiritual force. Our true purpose is not to be selfish but to serve others. Selfishness is not of our spirit, it's from our weak ego. We transcend this ego weakness by having compassion for each other through the love of our spirit. In order to complete this important spiritual step we may need to eliminate our own personal emotional waste, just as our body naturally eliminate its waste. We must first complete ourselves as individuals. Then we're ready to be collectively connected in the spirit.

SELF ACCEPTANCE and CONTROL EQUALS WEIGHT CONTROL

Accepting ourselves as we are right now, is our best approach. Self-acceptance transcends the need for everyone else's acceptance of us. If one of our fears is that people won't accept us as we are, we need not worry about that. Once we have accepted ourselves, people will accept us also. Valuing ourselves is really what matters. By accepting ourselves, we can share our best self with others. This will reinforce our own self acceptance and allow us to control and love ourselves completely. This is also when other people appreciate us the most because we're genuine. In my desire for a healthy and fit physique I had to think big, bold, and positive. Although I have not reached the pinnacle of all my goals, it is for that challenge that I go on. My daily gains in positive self-worth and self-love brings me happiness. When we accept who we are, we obviate the need to simulate worthiness. The more we grow and learn, the more we can live life abundantly. Knowing our life's purpose is the only way to improve the quality of our lives. Knowledge is good. It makes the adventure through life more manageable. Our weight loss and fitness goals can be achieved through the magnitude of our motivation and the power of our knowledge working in unison. However, be mindful that knowledge without action is worthless. Persistence is also key here. We may fall ten times as a heavy weight. But as long as we get up for the eleventh round, we will be a lighter-weight champion. We can only measure the dept of our accomplishments by the adversities we overcome. The truth is there will be a myriad of adversities to overcome, but their purpose is to build our physical muscles as well as build our spiritual muscles. It is in our sharing of such adversities that we can connect socially, mentally and eventually spiritually. The only requirement is that our intent be deeply authentic.

Facing Fear Of Failure With Positive Self-Talk and Taking Charge

Like a snake, we can make that permanent and positive change in our health and fitness, never to return to our old skin. To be winners, we must confront our fear head-on; that's half the battle. Fear is not a brick wall. We can walk through our fear. We can do this by asking ourselves "what if" questions. For example: What if I don't fit into my wedding dress; can I lose weight for my wedding? Can I get fit for life? Will I be healthy again? So what if I just had a baby, and I am sixty pounds overweight? Would losing it make me healthier, happier, and more confident? If you answered "yes," to a least two of these questions then please take action. Weight loss is not an overnight event, but you can get mentally ready today. Becoming a beginner will **make us winners**.

Getting started and sticking with the program is what self-empowerment, and taking change is all about. We need not kill ourselves with brute force for shallow gains; or become a weekend warrior. But instead stay focused and persistent. Diligence is the beauty of good luck, we make our own luck diligently. A weapon that is more powerful than luck is still called pro-action. It is in our doing that we become confident.

We may ask, "How do I develop confidence?" My answer to

that is: "We start at our present level—where we are now. If we need to lose fifty pounds, we start by setting small goals. Lose one solid pound first, and keep climbing the mountain until you reach the top.

Solid Goals are The Path To Our Desire

We must set goals great enough to matter and small enough to do. First, spend quiet time with yourself to become familiar with the landscape of your desires. Then clearly identify in your mind the goals you'd like to attain. Secondly, crystallize your purpose with your goals, and move forward. Your main purpose should always be to be healthy, happy, and at peace with your self. Set lifetime goals, not quick fixes. Choose goals you know will greatly improve the quality of your life and that are easy enough for you to handle. It may be to give up one junk food item per day, say a candy bar or a bag of chips. If you can't handle that every day do it every two days. When you're able to handle cold turkey every two days, try it every other day until you overcome. Forget about feeling unworthy of anything good that you want for yourself. Being alive makes us all worthy of being healthy, wealthy, and wise. Our lives have purpose, but in order to fulfill that purpose we must be in good health, body, mind, and soul. A regular practice of selflessness is another way to replace the craving of junk food, as well as to relieve stress in our lives. We can try giving away some of our time or our money. We can become a mentor for a child, a volunteer for meals on wheels, or work for a homeless shelter. Reaching out is godly. It boosts our energy level, and it's constructive exercise that strengthens our immune system. Giving of ourselves is a way of saying we have more than we need; we are blessed, and others are worthwhile. One principle that will help us to live life more abundantly is to build our self-confidence, by doing for someone less fortunate. Such small goals are greater than gold to somebody, and it adds years of happiness to our lives. Doing good deeds is one of the best stress relievers. Whatever good we donate to the universe will be returned ten-fold. In fact, some of our JFJ cravings are really a symptom of not reaching out to others in a positive way.

Every little goal that we've reached makes us all winners. The important thing is that we did it. Sometimes that's the emotional food we need to fill the emptiness inside of us. Just imagine if we all set and met little goals every day! Picture all of us women sowing little seeds of new and improved habits. The possibilities would be unlimited. The old proverb said, "Sow a thought reap an action, sow an action, reap a habit; sow a set of habits, reap a character; sow a character, and reap your destiny." WOW! This is how we can complete our connection to self and others.

How to Sow Thoughts that will Erase Negativity and Build our Confidence with Positive Mental Potions

Confidence Builders (CB's) are necessary because our lives are completely dominated by our thoughts. Whatever our minds bring on the screen, our bodies will gravitate towards. When we think of junk food all day, we end up eating them. When we think about the JFJ, we end up there. Yes, our will are broken by our own negative thoughts because they lead us into temptation and negative actions. A daily dosage of positive thoughts, and energy followed by positive actions will build unshakable confidence. Imagining ourselves eating healthful foods and exercising regularly will lead us to change our diet and join a gym. All great events or works of art began with an inspiration, a picture in someone's mind, followed by a leap into action. Because our moods can be controlled through our thoughts, we must command when and what we think. I have become very skilled in dismissing negativity from my mind. I quickly ask myself, "Will this thought bring me peace?" If a big *No* jumps at me, I gently dismiss the thought; this action has brought me much inner peace. Let's begin to meditate upon the following positive mental potions until they sink into our unconscious mind and become a part of our automatic thinking.

"I erase all doubts and fears from my consciousness."
"I will manifest my desires."
"I am willing to transcend myself beyond my current reality of stress."

" I will learn how to make stress a friend."
"I will not get lost in the junk food jungle."
"I don't have to be overweight, and out of shape for any reason." "I still want to feel attractive, healthy, fit, and yes, beautiful!"
"As women, we must believe in ourselves always, especially when no one else does."
"We must take responsibility for our present position in life, never surrender leadership and never give control of our lives to others."
"Don't blame other people for your shortcomings or mistakes in life. Admit them readily."

My feeling is that we become what we think about most. I became a successful body-builder because I thought about getting back into shape. I acted on my thoughts, and it took me further than I could imagine possible! I'm not a competitive body-builder anymore, nor do I care to be. Bodybuilding helped me to connect to my spirit, which allowed me to enjoy a beautiful and healthy body. It also helped to speed up the process of exercising good discipline. Think of your ability to change bad thoughts as a remote control. When negative thoughts arise — change your channel or go for a walk instead.

We must remind ourselves that we can not become what we need to be by remaining what we are now. We are to see our daily problems as daily practice towards improvement.

1. We must rehearse mentally every day.

2. Be a believer and act as if our dreams will happen.

3. We must downplay our fears and success will favor us.

4. We will be a size 12, 10, 8, or 5 (or whatever size we want to be) again if we deeply believe this; it's called faith.

5. Use the words if I think I can't or if I think I can - I'm right. The truth is you can. Whatever we believe we can manifest when we concentrate, meditate, or pray on it.

6. When we are sold on our desires, we must not doubt ourselves, but we must take action.

7. A) Have courage, B) Take chances, and C) Take control.

8. We have nothing to lose except maybe a few pounds of fat. Have faith but don't give in to fate by thinking, "That's my lot in life, I can't change a thing, I'll always be fat." Rubbish. We can keep outside influences at bay, and go within. After all, we know ourselves best.

We can get in touch with our needs and wants, shape our own body and our own destiny, by making wise decisions. After every wise decision, we must follow up with immediate action. My mother always say "time waits for no man, and it changes nothing, when we do nothing", the truth is we actually have to make changes ourselves. I say when it comes to our lives "WE" definitely should not wait for time to do it for us, it will never get done this way. We cannot afford to drift through life in a daze; challenges will confront us, and face them we must. Never give in to adversity, and never give up your dreams. Our dreams are usually our purpose in life. Even when we feel discouraged about our dreams, whatever they are, keep moving towards them. Most of us end up in despair, because we've lost track of our dreams. A person without a dream is like a ship without a rudder, destined for nowhere. We should take regular inventory of the quality of our lives. We need to look inside into our souls and evaluate the conditions. Women tend to look outside of themselves for answers. We usually get stuck trying to find answers, get permission, get advice, and get approval from outside. We all need each other sometimes but it is wise to know whom and to know when. We're all sisters in love, if not in law, but we need to give each other the space to seek and to find ourselves first. Society's image of women's beauty is strong, but we must overcome them with good sense, and personal power, and move forward. We know what's best for us, therefore, we must measure our standards based on our individual potential. Keeping up with the Jones is mindless. We must always be mindful of our own deep purpose and destiny. We rob ourselves of our happiness when we make comparisons of ourselves to other people. For example, when we believe we fall short or are inferior in comparison to super models and blonde beauties on TV, on billboards, in movies, and in glamour magazines. The only person we need to compare ourselves to is our own self as we watch ourselves become better and better every day.

Don't Worry, Be Healthy

As a nurse I have seen people try to destroy themselves via stress overload, eating disorders such as anorexia, drinking, smoking, drug abuse, starving the body during pregnancy, bingeing and purging, or just plain overeating themselves to the point of fatality. These are all extremes of decadent compulsive behaviors. We don't have to be labeled anorexic, bulimic, or obese to have an eating disorder. Most of us would agree that an immediate snack would pacify our psyche when we're stressed. But long-term it leads us into severe stress, depression, and an eating disorder. Most of us are diet junkies or nutritional neurotics. We simultaneously lust after leanness, while we crave the cheesecake. Most of us succumb to the temptation because we want to have our cake and eat it, too. So, none of us can wag a finger. We all have an eating disorder to some degree. A wise approach to successful weight control and beauty is to be honest with ourselves. By taking baby steps at a time, we can inch our way to health; inch by inch any waist line is a cinch.

It's not wise to compare our waistline to any visual images we see in public.

We are to erase our childhood fantasies of glamour and get real. If we need to grow up, let's do it together, so we can teach our daughters wisely. We do not wish for them to become future anorexics. The average woman weighs 130 pounds and is five foot, three inches tall. The average woman gets pregnant and has babies, and we know what comes along with that. For all the young women who haven't had kids yet, let me spell it out for you and for all you moms, *pregnancy is a beautiful life-giving process*. It is truly our lifeline, if not for pregnancy none of us would be here. I respect and honor my mother for having me. On the other hand, there are price tags attached. Pregnancy is taxing on our bodies, our health, physical fitness, appearance, and sexuality. We gain weight along with gaining the baby. We lose sleep, and we lose some of our sex life, but in the end, we have created a life, and that is worth the hassle. Remember that as long as we still have life, we still have hope. Can we survive all of that, and bounce back? Absolutely, positively, yes, we **CAN**. We are the ***women being***. Mother Nature has blessed us with this gift. I've done it for the past sixteen years. There is nothing different about me. We're just at different stages in our lives. I've reached my goal and am now maintaining and holding. You could be on your way, too. If you're going to do it, it's up to you. Wise women model themselves after successful women. They do not re-invent the wheel. You've got all the help you need to get started in the palms of your hands. Now is the time to log on the screen and change your self-image.

Chapter 3

Dispelling the Myths About Diet, Nutrition, Surgical Procedures and Permanent Weight Loss

In this chapter we will explore the following:.
- Good Nutrition Can Enrich And Pep-Up our Lives.
- Nutritional Control vs. Weight Control.
- Don't Get Distracted.
- Taste Is Our Servant Not Our Master.
- Valuing Nutrients Over Taste.
- What Is Good Nutrition.
- Basic Nutritional Concepts.
- Beyond Willpower.
- Temptations Of The Senses.
- How Good Are Goodies?
- Making Willpower Work For Us.
- Eating Disorders

Maybe you're clueless as to what's sabotaging your weight loss efforts. Perhaps you've tried many times to lose weight only to lose a few pounds and gain a lot more in the end.

If you are like most people, you probably have a few misconceptions or myths about your dietary habits. These myths can deprive you of experiencing maximum health. Maybe your diet needs a little streamlining which could make a drastic improvement in your everyday energy level, your enthusiasm, passion for living, and your ultimate enjoyment and quality of life.

First, let's take a look at the dieting patterns that dominate most women in America. Without much thought, some of us are our own worst enemies. For example, we often get sidetracked by trends such as fad diets or diet pills that keep us undernourished. Or we may do the opposite, we go on " see food diets," eating everything in sight and becoming overweight. Some of us alternate between conforming and nonconforming as we watch our bodies inflate and deflate, flip, flop, and flab away. Some of us are obsessed with trying new recipes. Some that are so good they're bad for our health. In America, the major problem with food is not the scarcity of it. It's the abundance of rich gourmet and/or junk foods and the over-consumption of these foods that is killing us. These foods are drained of their natural nutrients, and are loaded with fats, cholesterol, and chemicals. They lead us into the path of high cholesterol, diabetes, obesity, and various cardiac diseases. The news now reports that twelve-year-olds and teenagers are being diagnosed with Type-2 adult diabetes. Our bodies are constantly at war, just battling to survive each snack attack or nutritional insult. As a nurse I have seen American women wander into the hospital, wearing the years of their diets on their hips as a ring around the waist. These women are the unfortunate turtles in the horse race of health in this age of enlightenment. This is not a moral judgment, however. It is my professional observation of the ugly facts that most of us would like to ignore. Facts I feel I am obligated to bring to light. We are all players in the game of good health on this planet, and we must acknowledge that we take full responsibility for this result. Apparently, we are concerned more with the pleasure of eating and less often with the benefits of what we eat. Some of us are truly not aware of the great powers of good nutrition. We need to get "value" from what we eat. Our daily bread is the backbone of our future health. Without that support structure, we will perish in the JFJ. Onlookers always have a grimace on their faces when they see my green drink. They're more concerned about its taste than its nutritional content. "How does it taste?" is always the question. The nutritional content is of far less interest. Similarly, pleasurable foods are usually a liability to our health and well being. This is unfortunate, because many highly nutritious foods are also delicious. This is a valuable message to get across to our kids before they get trapped in the seductive junk food jungle.

Good Nutrition Can Enrich and Pep-Up our Lives

Positive and productive changes in our nutritional lifestyles can give us pep and something to look forward to. Good nutritional habits are our personal insurance policies against being overweight, enduring poor health, suffering diseases, malnutrition, stress, and premature death.

Most of the women I have worked with have had bad experiences dabbling with diets. They would lose weight, then gain the weight back plus an additional five to fifteen and sometimes more, pounds. Sooner or later they realized that their weight loss crash/fad diets were destructive, and counter-productive. Their prolonged attempts at trying to lose weight, and failing again and again, resulted in both physical and mental anguish. This is stress at its best, a hard battle to fight without the proper tools. I can sympathize with this struggle, but there is hope and a lot of help in the rest of this book. One approach to learned helplessness for some women is to surrender themselves to the gods of the JFJ. When we're overwhelmed with stress, our bodies and minds will protest, which is why we resort to desperate measures without thinking them through.

Out of desperation, some women have resorted to other alternatives or various surgical procedures, such as: stomach reduction, stapling their mouth shut, tummy tucks, or lipo-suction. We do know those surgical procedures and quick fix diets are not ideal for proper weight loss and good health; therefore they are not healthful long-term solutions. It is usually our bruised ego, or low self-image, that craves attention. In order to mask our feelings of desperation, we seek immediate treatments to avoid our pain and responsibility. For some women, this decision can be harmful, or even deadly.

We are more obsessed with how lipo-suction will make us look than we are with the dangers of the surgery. We minimize the risks involved, and we magnify the promises, however, unrealistic they may be. It is human to want an easy way out of difficult situations.

However, let us use caution. In some cases lipo-suction has been an asset. The look is great for a while, but, ultimately, we have to make a real change in our lifestyle. For instance, if one gets lipo-suction but still continues to eat everything in sight, the problem is going to come back. The down side of lipo-suction is that many women have been disappointed with their surgical results.

Some of them have had nightmare procedures that have disfigured them for life. Selecting a board certified cosmetic surgeon is paramount. While surgeons and their surgical procedures can be a dangerous gamble, proper nutrition and exercise, along with stress reduction, are always safe and appropriate for every one. Fad diets and surgery does not prevent killer diseases such as high cholesterol, heart disease, and cancer; they do not make us physically fit or healthy, either. The success of our health is still hidden behind persistent wise actions. The safest way to lose weight is still the old fashioned way by maintaining a proper low-fat diet coupled with daily exercise. These measures promote overall good health, not just thinness. I am not against surgery. I just think it should be a last resort unless medically indicated. Surgery is not the whole enchilada. Cardiac fitness, weight stabilization, physical endurance, mental health, and happiness are more important than a thin appearance. Utilizing our newfound knowledge here can help us to reframe and change our destructive behaviors. We live in a stimulus response world, but when it comes to our health it is prudent to respond with wisdom and to model after successful people. They always leave footprints in the sand for us to follow.

Nutrition Control vs. Weight Control

Let's begin this discussion with the concept of "positive healthful nutrition." Coming up is a quick quiz to test your nutrition IQ. Do you practice good nutrition? Whatever your score is you can upgrade it by increasing your knowledge of nutrition. Use this guide as a baseline to judge your present eating habits.

Do you awake feeling grateful to be alive?
Are you mostly in a good mood?
Are you motivated to get the best out of your day?
Are you committed to eat a healthful diet one-day at a time?
These "attitudes" can add years to your life and life to your years. Adopt them as your own!

Nutrition Quiz (Answer: Yes, No, or Sometimes)
- Do you desire to live a healthy lifestyle?
- Have you willingly chosen to make changes in your diet?
- Are you ready to empower yourself and take posi-

tive action towards good health?
- Do you eat breakfast everyday?
- Do you eat regular meals?
- Do you eat at the same time for each meal?
- Do you drink decaffeinated coffee?
- Or just have one or two cups of regular coffee?
- Do you limit or avoid table sugar?
- Do you always avoid eating greasy and salty fast-foods?
- Do you avoid adding salt to your food?
- Do you avoid eating red meat or eat very little of it?
- Do you avoid eating egg yolks or eat them only occasionally? (The egg white is ok)
- Do you avoid fats, butter, margarine, mayonnaise, oils, high-fat salad dressings, and high-fat dairy products, such as whole milk, cheese, ice cream, and excess cream in coffee?
- Do you read labels to avoid foods that are high in preservatives, sugar, fat, and salt?
- Do you consume four or more servings of fruits (or fruit juices) and vegetables daily?
- Do you consume whole grains, legumes, and fiber?
- Do you have at least 2-3 glasses of plain water a day?
- Do you sleep through the night without waking for a snack?
- Do you keep negative thoughts at bay?
- Do you take responsibility for your mistakes readily?
- Do you keep your days as stress-free as possible?

If you have answered yes to all or most of these questions, your nutritional habits are in great shape. If you answered **no or sometimes** to any or many of these questions, you need to examine your nutritional life-style and make some changes. As responsible adults we have to make an effort to avoid our sugar and spice and various vices from our food intake. Yes! We need a mute button to silence the screams of the junk food jungle.

We cannot continue to live by the law of anything that can go wrong will. That thought could destroy our day. Here is a better law to contemplate first thing every morning, if we can make it go right we will.

Don't Get Distracted

Because our thoughts rock our world, we must be focused, especially since we have to face the junk food jungle every day of our lives. All five of our senses are being triggered every minute of our waking day, in the biggest stimulus response laboratory for humans called the junk food jungle. Our nutrition, good or bad, will affect us, both physically and emotionally. On one hand we must eat to survive, our bodies need food as much as it needs air and water. These basic life support materials give our body the essential chemicals and energy that enable us to function. On the other hand, food has many emotional strings attached. They can be personal, cultural, or social. Although food and water are essential for survival, we do not sustain our physical bodies merely by the mechanics of mere eating. We attach our emotions to particular foods. I guess that's why almost all of my patients complained to me about the hospital food being lousy or that they don't have an appetite, or insist that they can't wait to go home for some good, old-fashioned cooking. Mom or grandma's cooking is always the best. It has magical powers that can heal our hearts and our souls. This is why home is where the heart is. This is also why we need to learn how to care for, and love, our hearts right there in our own homes. Before our hearts, and our kids' hearts, become attached to the killer foods, let's cut the fat, lower the sugar, and prevent the blues.

Taste as our Servants, not our Master: Valuing Nutrition over Taste

We all need to develop a practical application of nutrition. We can educate ourselves and use the knowledge we gain to combat malnutrition and misinformation. We need to open our minds, and change our attitudes about food. We need to begin to think of food as preventive medicine. We must first ask ourselves, "Is the food healthful?" A big change that I made was to learn to value nutrition over taste. The same way I try on a suit to see how well it fits is the same way I think about how each food item will look on me, and in me, before I consume it. The questions I ask myself are: "Will this make me healthier? Will it bring me closer to what I want to look like? Will it give me more energy? Will I feel good about myself, or will I feel guilty? Will this make me fat or fit? Is this food from the junk food jungle? Will my action bring me peace, or guilt?" Remember, I talked about making associations that link pain and obesity to junk foods and pleasure and looking good to healthful foods. Without the bitterness of adversity, prosperity wouldn't taste so good. Without natural foods, health wouldn't feel so good. The knowledge of nutrition has always steered me in the right direction. Do likewise; quit your membership to the junk food jungle and join my health club. Exercise your knowledge, and power. Take action now. The only powers behind our knowledge are the actual actions we take. If we take no action, we have no power for the long haul. **TAKE ACTION, LADIES!**

What is Good Nutrition?
Basic Nutritional Concepts

Good nutrition is our body's mighty army of defense against diseases, depression, and death by default.

1. Nutrition is what we eat and how our bodies utilize it.
2. The purpose of nutrition is to sustain life.
3. Nutrition also sustains health, energy, growth, and repair.
4. A combination of foods can provide a balanced diet.
5. No single food has all the nutrients needed for good health.
6. Each nutrient has a specific need by the body.
7. Nutrients work best when combined with others.
8. All individuals throughout life need the same nutrients in different proportions.
9. Gender, age, size, activity level, and health status influence nutritional needs.
10. The handling and preparation of food influence its nutritional content, appearance, and taste.
11. Handling is everything that happens to food during its growth, processing, storage, and preparation. An example of this is the addition of vitamins (fortification), chemicals,

and preservatives. Some of these chemicals can be carcinogenic and can contribute to various types of cancers.
12. Foods should be consumed, ideally, while they are still wholesome and fresh.
13. Foods should be combined, rotated, and taken from the basic food sources.
14. Our food intake should be the first source of disease prevention and health promotion.
15. Food should also be our fighting force against stress.
16. The restorative powers of nutrition can give us a new lease on life.
17. Our health is usually an expression of what we think about, and what we eat.
18. Total health is a continuum of our body, mind, and spirit. A healthy body creates a healthy mind and spirit.

Beyond Willpower

Willpower cannot keep us thin for long. It ironically leads us down the avenue of powerlessness. In fact, it's a misconception that we can achieve by suppressing our urges with brute force of will. Most people are not able to will their powers long enough to sustain permanent weight loss. To rely on willpower is to add tremendous stress to our lives BMS. Willpower is often unfairly linked to weight loss. Society at large seems to think that the secret of weight loss success is to have willpower, especially when it relates to behavioral changes such as dieting. We see an overweight person and automatically stereotype that person as someone with "no willpower." It is true that willpower is a great motivator and an expression of one's strength of character. However, willpower is also like a car battery that gradually dies. Willpower is not enough to maintain a person on a successful weight loss and maintenance program. It is not enough to keep us through the long haul of life. When people fall off their diets and exercise wagons, they immediately assume that it was their lack of willpower that failed them. This type of thinking is self-defeating. When we tell our subconscious that we have no power we will gradually accept failures in our lives. The degree to which we accept failure is to the same degree that we will fail. My feeling is that willpower is only a small part of our potential. Depending on willpower alone tends to make weight loss a moral issue. We must not be distracted by others, but instead, stick to our own wisdom and spiritual counsel. When we're in need of strength we can always find it if we have the courage to look within and search our own heart. Our personal health is just for us. It's not to convince others or **"to show them."** This attitude is more of a self-inflicted stress that only serves to weaken our will and grieve our spirit. We must keep our ego out of this equation before we trip on it. There is no room for self-righteousness in a program of healthy living. What we want is inner peace and relaxation, not self-inflicted stress. Healthy living is a matter of what's right for us. ***True willpower is making wise decisions and acting on them readily.*** It's our choice to keep ourselves empowered and to take charge of our own health. We must not pass judgment on ourselves or in other people. Until we walk a mile in someone else's shoes, let us reserve judgement, even if that someone is our self. If we choose to lose weight on willpower alone, we will most likely fail. When we do fail, we're worse off than when we first started. Being human, our pride may get in the way of trying again, and we may want to give up. In this case, ego and pride are always the enemies. We must put them aside, lick our wounds, and move forward with our fitness goals relying on the strength of our spirit to sustain us. We can do this by diligently building our ability one step at a time. Building that ability requires no prior skill. We need not expend excess energy to keep going to impress others. We humbly build on our daily progress period. We must not quit until we escape the junk food jungle, physically as well as mentally. Sometimes the mental temptations are the biggest hurdles to overcome. Because we can only harbor one thought at a time, let us focus on positive outcomes such as: **good health, and a prosperous purpose for our future.**

Temptations Of The Senses

When faced with temptations: how can we zip our lips and pretend we can't taste? Shut our eyes and pretend we're blind? Plug our ears and pretend we're deaf? Stop breathing and pretend we can't smell? And stop swallowing and pretend we can't feel the texture of foods? Today it's a jungle out there, and we still struggle with the stress of sensory perception and temptations. The junk food jungle is so intoxicating. Its smells are seductive. Its sight is captivating. Its taste is addicting and its textures are seductive. With only one bite of the junk food jungle we could be hooked. Our entire course of action could lead to destruction. Yielding to temptation can be a big mistake in more ways than one. How many times, and in how many ways, can we overdose in the jungle and survive? That's a question nobody knows the answer to, but we continue to be tempted by the serpents of **the junk food jungle**.

These temptations are well calculated by advertisers. All they need is thirty seconds to grab our sensitive nerve and pull until we say ok. For example: consider the all-you-can-eat deals, buy one and you will get one free. These are all ways to tempt consumers into purchasing foods that are like wolves in sheep's clothing. One of my female clients told me that she could not resist a good food bargain. She took her kids to all the fast food specials. On weekends, she went for the *all you can eat specials* at a restaurant. Her favorite was the Sunday brunches, the dessert section. She also said (with a grin on her face), "I would make sure that I got my money's worth too, by really eating all that I could eat." She was a forty-six-year-old homemaker who had a lot of time on her hands. She said, "When my kids are in school, I call up my girlfriends and tell them about the specials. Then I would ask them to go to lunch with me." Because of that, she really didn't lose her weight after each pregnancy. She just continued to gain weight. This woman was completely obsessed with food. Her every moment in life was driven by the thought of food. About 250 pounds, and 5 feet 4 inches tall, she continued to grow horizontally. She came to see me with a determination, and a blazing desire to take charge of her life. She wanted to know what healthful eating was about. She had a few private consults with me. She learned how to eat and exercise properly and has been slowly losing fat as she continues to take charge of her nutrition and exercise regimen. [So called-Lucille] now has confidence in herself and in her ability to take charge. I think [Lucille] speaks for a lot of overweight people who struggle with the cultural temptations of our junk food jungle.

There is a way to keep temptation at bay and that is to keep ahead of it. If you are concerned that you might stop at the ice cream parlor on your way to pick up the kids, drive home another way. Now is the time to go down the tunnel without the cheese. After all, we are not really rats. Take an apple with you in the car and have that before you become tempted to stop at a junk food store. Be vigilant, be prepared, and be pro-active. I always take a fruit snack with me; it gives me a biting chance. If you do this often enough, you will break the bad habit and replace it with a healthful one. Every time we weaken the power of a bad habit, we should also reinforce a good habit.

How Good Are Goodies?

We all know the answer to this question. Goodies are usually good enough for some of us to have seconds, and thirds, or just to constantly pick and nibble for the sheer pleasure of indulging our taste buds. But remember taste buds are our servants. We can train them to **"RESPECT"** the taste of healthful foods. The constant pecking, and pleasuring, of our taste buds is frightening, because we lose track. Most of us gain weight this way. After a while, nibbling becomes automatic. A significant number of calories can be consumed while nibbling, with no consciousness of our actions. At the same time, nibbling can mean that we remain hungry, unsatisfied, and deprived of a proper meal. In the end, we're still hungry. We may fantasize or think about how great certain foods taste and how we desire to eat them. We often unconsciously condition ourselves to respond to our thoughts of food. We induce a hunger response in ourselves. That is why it is important to nibble only on healthful, non-fat, nutritious snacks. They kill our cravings, do us no harm, and are a benefit to our health. In humans, the cerebral cortex and the limbic system respond to thoughts unconsciously (this may be called unconscious response to external stimulation). When we see, smell, or fantasize about foods, the limbic system responds involuntarily by increasing our salivation. This is a response that prepares the body for digestion. It thinks that we're going to eat. The body has trouble separating the thought from the actual behavior. In addition to our mouth watering, insulin will be released into the blood; this lowers blood sugar and causes us to feel hungry. At this point, we may overindulge, feeling justified that we were hungry when, in fact, we have unconsciously induced our own hunger by falling prey to the stimulus response syndrome. If we choose not to eat, the drive to eat will persist (what we try to resist will persist). Our body could compensate by breaking down muscles for energy (in order to stabilize our blood sugar level). If we eat after triggering a hunger response, most of what we eat will be stored as fat. Whenever the body experiences a low blood sugar, the body protects itself by storing the foods that are being consumed at that point as fat, because it thinks it is being starved. The fluctuation in blood sugar informs the body that there is a famine coming, which leads the body to protect itself from its presumed starvation, by being defensive. The female body's defensive mechanism to starvation is to crave fat, and store fat just in case we get pregnant. Our body is preparing for its purpose in nature. As a result of this artificial stimulation of hunger, we often end up eating when we are really not hungry. The average person gets hungry at four-hour intervals, give or take an hour. The frequency of hunger depends on one's age, sex, activity level, individual metabolism, level of health, and the amount, time, and type of the last meal. Humans can also trigger the response for food digestion at the stimulation of our senses, i.e. sight, smell, taste, touch, and feel of foods. These unconscious responses happen quickly before we're able to consciously realize that we really shouldn't be hungry at that particular time because we have already had a good breakfast or lunch an hour ago or we quickly forget that we had a healthful dinner planned for the evening. This is another case of negative association affecting when and what we eat. This knowledge of our unconscious responses should make us more aware of our thoughts about foods and inspire us to think healthful thoughts about foods. This is another way of saying that the thoughts we feed our minds are just as important as the food we feed our bodies.

CONNECTION COMPLETE

Making Willpower Work for Us

The most important message I hope to get across in this chapter is that willpower will not be enough to keep us from being tempted or from yielding to temptation. Relying on willpower alone will lead us to deprivation, sometimes even depression, from not being able to satisfy our food fantasies. This is a catch-22 situation. We pay if we eat junk foods by gaining weight. Alternatively, if we starve ourselves, we pay the price of losing muscle mass, because our bodies will begin to break down skeletal muscle for energy whenever it's being deprived. The balance between these two situations is to maintain a healthy diet and keep our blood sugar levels stable. Willpower is only powerful when it's combined with knowledge, discipline and planning. These qualities will get us through the rough times until our bodies become adjusted to the new discipline. As we practice our new, healthy habits, we will gradually become less interested in junk foods. We'll be more turned on to how great we're beginning to look and feel, and that's the best motivation of all. Just a word of encouragement: It is sacrificial to make essential changes in our nutritional life styles. Nevertheless, we must keep at it. We're worth it. Don't give up. We also shouldn't feel that we're weak or a failure when we get tempted or when we succumb to temptation. We need to give ourselves credit for the ***honest efforts*** we make. None of us are perfect therefore we need not judge ourselves too harshly. Our judgment of ourselves is more self-destructive than productive.

If you happen to indulge in unhealthful eating, just acknowledge it and get back on the right track. We need not flog ourselves with words of woe. We can pull up our anchors of agony and begin to advance in the right direction. We might want to give a pseudonym to the cheater in us. When we decide to cheat, we can look into the mirror and tell "Jane," to get out of our lives, to leave us alone, because we don't like what she is doing to our bodies. As long as we're willing to stick to our **goals**, the power of our **WILL**, will work. ***Remember: Willpower is about actions taken and perseverance, not perfection.*** Most often it is when we make a mistake or we fall down that we learn to stand up and become stronger.

Eating Disorders

The ability and drive to control one's weight and health are viewed as power tools. It is popular to be body conscious and lean. Dieting and exercising to maintain fitness is great, but compulsive starvation to be thin or compulsive dieting and exercising to cover up compulsive eating is threatening to our health, sometimes even to our lives. Could it be that your teenager, or even you or your child, is a dieting anorexic or an exercising bulimic? These disorders are affecting women of all ages today; it's almost a cradle-to-the-grave syndrome. Here are some questions for you:

1. *Does concern about your weight govern your lifestyle?*
2. *Does the scale control your mood and your daily schedule?*
3. *Do you have regular nightmares of being a fat, out-of-control person?*
4. *Are you obsessed with eating, exercising, or starving yourself?*
5. *Are you a binger or purger?*
6. *Are you a chronic dieter who is underweight but you think you look fat?*
7. *Are you obsessed with food?*
8. *Are you obsessed with your body image?*
9. *Do you constantly look in the mirror, or do you avoid the mirror?*
10. *Are you stressed-out about your weight and appearance?*
11. *Are people mentioning that you have lost or gained weight?*
12. *Do you hate your body?*

If you're someone who has said yes to any of these questions, if you are the mother of a child having such problems or if you are a teenager reading this book, you need to seek more extensive clinical help right away. This book can help you but only in conjunction with hands on clinical monitoring from an eating disorder specialist. They will provide the appropriate individualized treatment, based on your clinical findings after a thorough medical exam. Once you've dealt with your eating disorder medically, this book will help you to choose and eat wisely in the future. You can do it. Your decision to take charge and do old things in new ways is the magic that will transform you. We must focus on our goals and not

CONNECTION COMPLETE

our pain. With such a focus, we'll find our path to be smoother, and the way is always up! Remember, knowledge is only potential power. It is only when we take positive action that we really exercise our authentic power. Make a decision, and act now! Our mission is to make it through the long haul in great health, BMS.

Chapter 4

Our Nutritional Umbilical Life Line

Protein, Fats, Carbohydrates, & Vitamins

In this chapter we'll discuss:
- Protein: Our Life Source
- Main Sources Of Protein
- Getting Enough Protein as a Vegetarian
- The Egg White is a Pristine Protein
- Fats: Friend Or Foe
- Fat Makes Fat, Saturated And Unsaturated Fats
- A Little Lube For Your Tube
- Carbohydrates Good, Bad And Ugly
- Protein Sparing Carbohydrate Actions
- Avoid Sugar and Processed Foods .
- Simple Carbohydrates
- Complex Carbohydrates
- Salt Consumption
- The Krebs Cycle
- Accentuate The Positive Traits of Foods

Proteins, fats, carbohydrates, salt, and water, are dictators of our weight/health. We'll be talking about how foods affect the body in ways you may never have thought of before. You will be able to make up your own menu and eliminate destructive foods from your life. You will understand how to follow a low-fat method of food selection and preparation that is necessary for proper nutrition and weight control.

Protein-OUR — Life Source

Protein is our body's most vital building material. It's the essential life-sustaining source for all growth, development, maintenance, and repair of tissue in our body. Protein is necessary for strength, vigor, and muscle building. Protein also builds blood, skin, bones, nerves, hair, and nails. Animal foods such as fish, milk, cheese, meat, and eggs contain large amounts of protein. Protein is also present in plant foods such as grains and legumes. Vegetable sources of protein may be incomplete proteins (not containing all the eight essential amino acids). Humans need 22 amino acids, eight of which are not produced by the body and must be consumed in the diet. These eight amino acids are called the eight essentials, or complete, amino acids. They are mostly found in dairy products, meat, fish, and egg whites. Our body's need for daily protein varies from individual to individual. Protein can be converted into carbohydrates as the body's energy source. This happens when there is a deficit in carbohydrate intake. However, excessive protein intake is damaging, it can overwork our kidneys in an effort to eliminate the excess protein. Each gram of protein yields four calories. Twenty grams of protein for the average adult per meal is ideal. However, the presence of any disease or illness will increase protein requirements. For example, after major surgery, the body uses more protein, and vitamin C to repair and rebuild tissue. Protein helps to prevent the blood and tissue fluids from becoming too acidic or too alkaline, thus stabilizes their pH. Athletes, especially bodybuilders, require a larger intake of protein. The U.S. Food and Drug Administration (FDA) recommends approximately one-gram of protein per kilogram of lean, body weight, daily, as an adult requirement. This can vary individually. It's also tricky because most people do not know their lean, body weight off hand; you may need to get tested.

Main Sources of Protein

I'm recommending that you try some of these ideas for protein. Fish is my favorite source of protein. I have fish almost every other day for lunch or dinner. Fish is low in fat and high in protein. Broiled salmon with lemon instead of butter is quite tasty. Tofu is also a good source of protein; low-fat tofu is available today. I sometimes have tofu with rice or in soups with vegetables. If you're worried about taste, here is a simpler way to have fun. Blend tofu with ice and fruits for a great, healthful drink. Tofu is excellent in cancer prevention. Broiled, baked, or grilled skinless chicken with lemon juice, vinegar, and a teaspoon of olive oil, seasoned to taste, is a regular Monday night dinner for me. Occasionally, I have a grilled turkey burger seasoned to taste. Last, but not least, is my regular lunch, canned white tuna packed in water. It's great with picante sauce and a salad.

Getting Enough Protein As a Vegetarian

Because vegetarians do not eat animal flesh they are more challenged in obtaining sufficient protein in their diet. The lacto-ova, who drinks milk and eats eggs has a easier job since both are complete proteins. The vegan, who does not drink milk or eat eggs has to be more creative in combining different sources of plant proteins.

Egg White is Pristine Protein

Separating the egg white from the yolk is a relatively new concept, but it's well worth doing. Forget the yolk, as it is high in cholesterol and fat. An egg yolk has 25-30 milligrams of cholesterol depending on its size. The body needs approximately 500 mg. of cholesterol per day. The egg white is a pure form of protein called albumen. It is one of the highest quality proteins; it is practically non-fat and non-cholesterol. An egg white is a complete protein. Remember you only need about 50 grams of protein per day. On average, as we age we need less and less protein. If you choose to have egg whites, you should know that each white is about six grams of protein, depending on the size of the egg. When I choose to blend my protein drink, I make sure that the eggs are not cracked; cracked eggs can cause salmonella poisoning. Egg whites are great if you're on the run—they're fast and easy to prepare. Boiled eggs can be easily separated. I usually separate three or four egg whites, add a splash of low-fat milk, then cook them in the microwave for two minutes. The milk keeps them nice and fluffy, but you need to stir after a minute. Then I sprinkle a pinch of salt and pepper or picante sauce on them to tickle my taste buds.

Fats: Friend or Foe

Fats are a concentrated energy source that is the last to be burned by the body but the first to be stored. Fats serve as fuel for energy, insulation, and protection for the internal organs of the body such as the heart and lungs. Society is becoming more and more aware of the need to reduce its excessive intake of saturated fats. Still, fat is a friend when helping the body to absorb vitamins A, E, K, and D, which are the fat-soluble vitamins. Fat also aids in the absorption of calcium to strengthen bones and teeth. Fat under the skin helps to retain heat and to stabilize body temperature. Each gram of fat yields nine calories. This is more than twice that of protein and carbohydrates, which is only four. The number one reason a high-fat diet results in fat storage is that individuals consume much more than they are able to burn. Excess dietary fats will always be stored. Don't let your abdomen appear before you do, cut the fat. The body prefers carbohydrates (CHO) to fat. It will burn CHO first. In many cases, fats are only metabolized after prolonged exercising, beyond two hours. You see why a low- or non-fat diet will prevent fat storage and weight gain. We also need our muscles in order to burn off fat. Some of my female clients were fat in spite of their regular exercises. They discovered (to their surprise) that it was their high-fat diets that were preventing their weight loss, as was true for me when I first started exercising. My skin was tight and firm, but not lean enough to show muscle definition, which was what I wanted. Once I discovered and discarded the hidden fats in my diet and consumed only non-fat dairy products, I started to lose body fat. My experience with the change in my diet was dramatic. I now know that the single most important change to make, in order to lose fat and to keep it off, is to cut fat out of the diet, or as much fat as possible. After all, we are human beings; we don't need to act as the squirrels do in storing fat (nuts) to get through the winter. In contrast, while they need their stored fat for their survival, we need to get rid of our stored fat for our survival.

Marcia Sheridan, R.N.

Fat Makes Fat: Saturated and Unsaturated Fats

Dietary fats are essentially saturated or unsaturated fats. Unsaturated fats are considered to be heart friendly. Unsaturated fats are of plant origin and are found in vegetables, seeds, grains, and nuts. Unsaturated fat is still fat. All sources of fat, saturated or unsaturated, can contribute to being overweight if eaten in excess. It is prudent to have small portions of nuts, seeds, and vegetable oils. Nature has more wisdom than we do and is a better judge of how much fat to yield in each vegetable to supply our needs.

The largest hidden source of calories in the diet is fat. Each fat gram has nine calories while proteins and carbohydrates have four calories. Saturated fats are usually solid at room temperature. Although coconut oil is liquid at room temperature, it is saturated. Saturated fats come from animal sources such as red meat, dairy products, and egg yolks. Saturated fats are linked to cardiovascular disease, obesity, colon cancer, breast cancer, and adult-onset diabetes. Saturated fats are a liability to our health and should be avoided. The largest hidden source of calories in the diet is fat. It is a challenge to keep saturated fat intake to 10 percent of our caloric intake but that would be ideal. There are disagreements here. Some say that's too low, but if you did it for a short intervals it would help more than it could possibly hurt.

A Little Lube for your Tubes
Linoleic Acid and Linolenic Acid

The daily requirement of the linoleic and linolenic fatty acids is one to two percent of our intake. These essential fatty acids are not produced by the body and are, therefore, necessary in the diet. They are found in sufficient amounts in beans, peas, vegetables, whole grains, and some fruits. These oils and fats are vital in making up the membranes that surround our cells. These cells are permeable meaning that they allow the passage of nutrients in and out of them. These fatty acids have other important functions, such as the absorption and transfer of fat-soluble vitamins and the good cholesterol, HDL, high-density lipoprotein. Linoleic acid helps to lower serum cholesterol through transport of cholesterol in our blood. This process helps to lower and keep our cholesterol down. It helps to strengthen cell membrane structure and capillaries. It also helps to prevent bleeding. By consuming natural foods, we won't run out of oil. It is important that we get oils from natural foods, because processed low-fat and non-fat foods are not reliable sources of essential oils (fatty acids). A lack of these essential oils can also contribute to heart disease and cancer.

Carbohydrates (CHO), Good Bad And Ugly

In order for life to go on, the body needs energy to perform. Carbohydrates are the main energy source for the human body, especially the brain. We need a daily dose to fire up our engines and keep us in operation all day; however, it must be high-octane premium. CHO can be derived mainly from fruits, plants, roots, yams, beans, pasta, brown rice, grains, and vegetables. Since the body can break down carbohydrates easier than it can fat and proteins to supply its energy needs, CHOs are called "quick energy foods." Remember that each gram of carbohydrate yields only four calories, while fat yields nine calories.

Protein-Sparing Carbohydrate Actions

Carbohydrates (CHO) help to regulate protein metabolism. Having sufficient CHO in the diet for energy demands will prevent the need for protein to be used to provide this energy. The protein-sparing action of CHO allows the major portion of our protein intake to build and repair tissues. The brain requires a minute-to-minute supply of CHO as its energy source. It has no stored supply of its own.

Although the brain does not store energy from CHO digestion, two other organs do for use in emergencies. CHO is stored as glycogen in the cardiac muscles and in the liver to be used when needed. This energy is released on demand such as times when the body is under stress and blood sugar is depleted. Athletes thrive on such energy storage. In addition to protein digestion, fat digestion is also aided by CHO intake. In order to burn fat, the body needs CHO to supply its energy source. Yes! It takes energy (calories) to burn fat. This is another reason why starvation diets do not promote fat burning. They do not give the body enough fuel (CHO) to work with. Fat only burns in the flame of CHO.

Processed Carbohydrates

Processed carbohydrates are exactly what they are called, processed. They are toxic to the body, and they make us ugly. Their nutritional value is poor, while they are loaded with chemicals and preservatives. Processed CHO are usually man-made goodies; for example, anything that is made with white sugar and white flour. The kind of foods that you see at a bake sale: cakes, cookies, pies, candies, and doughnuts are examples. These foods are also shocking to the blood sugar level. They will raise our blood sugar levels sky-high and trigger the onset of diabetes. They are not beneficial to the body. They yield empty calories and should not be highly consumed. They have an extremely high glycemic index, which means they are absorbed into the blood rapidly. This jolts our system like bolts of lightning. Some of us love these jolts, scientific findings. This is how we get the roller coaster effect in our blood sugar. One minute we feel like a racehorse and the next minute we feel like a turtle. The sugar high that we get is experienced after ingesting any sweet junk foods—such as candy, cake, or the like. The euphoric feeling we experience is very short-lived. As a reaction to very high blood sugar, the body releases insulin into the blood to buffer the high sugar into the cells in order to lower the blood sugar level. When our blood sugar is lowered so rapidly it causes us to experience a low feeling of fatigue, sleepiness, or a strong urge for another jolt. Pediatricians have learned, in their studies of hyperactive children, that sugar can be as addicting as nicotine/drugs. Be conscious. We must protect our children, as well as ourselves. Kids' hyperactivity has some direct relationship to their diet .

Avoid Sugar And Processed Foods

Experts have said that in one week, we consume the same amount of sugar our grandparents consumed in one year. Sugar is always present in manufactured foods. It's part of the preservation process. At one time or another, most of us get trapped in the blood sugar roller coaster ride. We call this a boost, but the cost is severe stress on our bodies. Appropriate intervention in diets (in most cases omission or reduction of sugar intake) can detoxify our systems of sugar. Some adult-onset diabetes can be exacerbated or triggered by a high intake of refined sugar. Susceptible individuals should conform to a low sugar diet and regular evaluation of their blood sugar levels. Blood sugar roller coaster rides can be rapid and deadly.

Simple Carbohydrates

Simple carbohydrates (meaning easy to digest) are natural sugars found mainly in fruits and some vegetables. Simple CHO require very little digestion and are quickly absorbed into the blood for energy. Simple CHO are what the human body is adapted to eat. Fruits are eighty to ninety percent water and contain most of the vitamin, mineral, and CHO requirements that the body needs. Simple carbohydrates have a low glycemic index. They stabilize blood sugar, unlike processed carbohydrates. Simple CHO pass through the stomach within minutes—with the exception of bananas which tend to take much longer. Fruits also release necessary enzymes and nutrients into the body. Fruits are best absorbed when eaten on an empty stomach. Have you ever noticed how an apple or pear takes the edge off your appetite? Therefore, fruits are an excellent choice as appetizers or for breakfast and they make for a great snack between meals. Having fruits in the mornings after a glass of water is a gentle way to warm up the gastrointestinal machine before a meal. Fruits also help to decrease acid indigestion and are a wonderful alternative to candy when we're craving sugar. The smell of a peach, an apple, a strawberry, or a mango is so calming. They make me anticipate the delightful experience to come. They lift our spirits and our blood level without bouncing us off the wall. Given this information, our intelligence quotient should draw us closer into the produce aisle. Combining different fruits is tasty and healthful. Here are some great choices: cantaloupe, tangerines, banana, apples, strawberries, pears, peaches, oranges, grapes, grapefruits, papaya, mangoes, and nectarines. Have more fruits; your body will love you for this, and you will love your body. In the old days, before vitamin tablets were invented, the vitamin C in limes allowed Britain to say goodbye to scurvy and hello to a great empire. Today our empire is our health. Let's build it one fruit at a time.

Complex Carbohydrates (CHO)

Complex CHO are more complex and require more time and work to be digested. They are the main source of our blood's energy supply. Complex CHO are supplied through vegetables, whole grains, beans, pasta, and roots. Complex CHOs provide a prolonged energy supply to the blood as they are broken down into simpler CHO. Complex CHO take a longer time (hours) to be completely digested; therefore, they stay in the stomach longer and prolong our sense of fullness, quite the opposite of (processed) refined CHO. Complex CHOs have a lower glycemic index compared to processed CHO. This means that they're absorbed smoothly and evenly into the blood. Complex CHO do not promote blood sugar fluctuations, "sugar blues" (cravings) and diabetic exacerbation. Complex CHO expand in the stomach and give a sensation of fullness that satisfies hunger for hours. Because we feel full, we are less preoccupied with food. Complex CHO also help us to be able to maintain control of our appetites. Complex CHO should be the chief source of energy for all body functions and muscular exertions. Complex CHO are actually the real food that our bodies are screaming for when we crave sugar. Complex CHO regulate protein and fat metabolism. Fats require CHO for their breakdown. Fats burn in the flame of carbohydrates as mentioned before. This is a major reason why there is no weight loss on a starvation diet. When the necessary carbohydrate intake is not available, there is nothing for the body to use as energy in order to burn fat. On the other hand, excess CHO in the diet will promote weight gain. Excess CHO will be converted into stored fat. Generally, it is better to have small portions of complex CHO as often as you feel hungry. Carbohydrates are friends that will help us to escape the Junk Food Jungle. They can be trusted to take us into health and happiness.

Salt Consumption

Let's talk a little about salt. Salt is one of the ingredients used in preserving and preparing foods in general. One of the biggest complaints I get from patients is that their food is too bland, "Not enough salt," they say. These people eat mostly foods that are very high in salt judging from their dietary history. They're the ones to reach for the salt shaker. Because the American diet is very high in salt, it contributes to a lot of diseases such as high blood pressure; which is due to water retention in the tissues that can cause circulatory congestion. This condition ultimately leads to heart disease as a result of the intense stress that is put on the heart to pump. Some of the other problems are swelling in the joints and stiffness, kidney disease, and just a tired, bloated feeling. Now can you see how one bad habit (salt shaking) can lead to disaster in slow motion? In this case, an ounce of prevention can save our health and longevity. Do we need salt? Yes! Everyone needs different amounts of salt intake. However, in America, there is no shortage of salt in the diet. The Food and Nutrition Board of the National Academy of Sciences considers a normal range of salt to be 1,100 to 3,300 milligrams per day. Compare that to the current estimate of daily intake of most adults which is 2,300 milligrams to 6,900 milligrams. As you can see, some people get over two to six times the amount they need in one day. Over the years this can be very dangerous to the heart and kidneys. Also, excess salt will cause water retention, especially in the feet. You may notice your feet are puffy and tightly fitting in your shoes, or your waist bursting out at the seams after a high salt meal or even after a bag of potato chips. The heavy hand on a salt shaker is equal to instant water weight and stress on our bodies. Most foods already have salt in them. We can get used to the natural taste of food by eating natural foods. Using less salt every day is a simple way to wean us from salt. It will take time to acquire that taste, but it will come. We must be strong and be the salt of the earth; but we need not eat more salt to do this. In fact, **LESS is MORE**.

The Krebs Cycle

The Krebs Cycle is the biochemical mechanism the body uses to burn calories. It's the melting pot of metabolism. All proteins, fats, CHO, and alcohol come together to be burned, recycled, stored, or modified, according to the body's needs. All that we eat is either stored as fat or burned for energy. When carbon and oxygen unite, carbon dioxide, water, and energy are given off. When we understand the Krebs Cycle, it can work in our favor. The Krebs Cycle, with some encouragement, will take us to the Promised body. It can turn more foods into substances such as carbon dioxide and water, which we exhale or excrete. With adequate water intake, the Krebs Cycle will be busy converting our CHO to carbon dioxide, water, and energy. These are usually excreted and burned off gradually within the activities of daily living. The Krebs Cycle does not produce water and store fat at the same time. It does one or the other at a given time. When we keep it busy making water and carbon dioxide, the fat-storing mechanism goes off because fat cells are being flushed with water. This will begin to shrink the size of each fat cell as they start to excrete water. The more fat cells we have, the more water weight we retain. Complex CHO, water and exercise, will burn our fat as our energy source. *(Remember: fat burns in the flame of CHO, and exercise, while protein will be spared to build and repair our muscles.)* If we do not take in enough CHO to aid in fat burning, our bodies will break down precious muscle tissues in order to provide the Krebs Cycle with the fuel it needs for energy. This is the worst thing we can allow to happen to us. Losing our muscles is like losing our minds. Having no tools to work with makes it impossible to reach our goals. You have just read about the properties, benefits, and the liabilities of foods we've known and have eaten for most of our lives. It's just a matter of shuffling them around like a deck of cards until we land a good hand. You are not expected to become an expert in nutrition after reading this chapter. You may even need to read it more than once. However, it is hoped that you will be able to use the information to your advantage. You will find that changing your diet is a long process and a lifetime commitment. Just keep your mantra in mind. We're in this for the long haul. We begin with education about the facts and then follow them along the path that will improve our health and quality of life. We also need to tap into our creative side for menu ideas that can please our palates, nourish our bodies, and boost our self-esteem. Above all, we must acknowledge the truth about our nutritional needs and decide to choose wisely.

Accentuate the Positive Traits of Foods

The real issue here is not just merely reading about fats, proteins, and CHO. It is also realizing how they can harm and how they can help us. Let's accentuate the positive for a moment. Imagine the possibilities if we took charge of our health with good nutrition and a healthful life style. We can eliminate the risks of heart disease, obesity, high blood pressure, and cancers. We can stop ourselves from becoming a statistic and a candidate for surgery, medicine, and an expensive hospital bed. We can also contact The American Heart Association and The American Dietetic Association for free brochures on heart healthy diets, health, and nutrition information. With the right information, we can make the changes that will help us leap into life-preserving life- styles. Even though our lives are our own individual journeys, we must plan to travel safely. All long journeys begin with a single step. We have taken that step, but we must keep on stepping along this well-chosen path until we escape the JFJ-body, mind, and soul.

Chapter 5

Why Fiber?

Fiber: The Backbone of our Diet

**Fiber is as important to our diet as
our digestive system is to our survival.**

Fiber gives the body a fighting chance against the JFJ. It's natures cleaning machine. It purges, rejuvenates, and restores order within our system.

- The virtues of fiber
- What is Fiber?
- Natural fiber supplements
- Diverticulitis and Discomforts, Stress To The Last Drop
- Fiber and Our Heart
- The Human Digestive System and Fiber
- Fiber As A Friend
- Fruits And Vegetables With Pectin
- Bran To The Rescue When We Cheat
- How To Increase Fiber In Our Diet
- Wok Cooking
- The Fiber Water Connection

The Virtues of Fibers

Allow me to open your mind just a little more on the virtues of fiber. Although there is an abundance of fiber in natural foods, the supply of fiber in the average American diet has steadily decreased because we have turned to refined, processed foods. Before the Industrial Revolution, the staple in our diet was fiber. This is not true today. Unfortunately, fiber has been replaced with nothing but processed/refined rubbish. For example, whole wheat is replaced by refined, white flour. Most families lived on farms. They cultivated their own food, which included potatoes, yams, beans, corns,

CONNECTION COMPLETE

fruits, and vegetables. These are all healthful, complex carbohydrates that are naturally rich in fiber. This lifestyle kept families physically active. People literally lived from the fat of the land. The kind of fat that kept us lean, mean, working machines. Their high physical activity coupled with their healthful bounty eliminated the need to add fiber to their diets. Today, people rely on pre-packaged foods. In our fast- paced, concrete jungle, we frequently eat on the run from a box or a plastic bag. Instead of fresh produce from our gardens, we race into the heart of the junk food jungle, only to get lost. But we do not notice this because we're more focused on the food than we are to the milieu. We can't see that we have left the land and are now in the junk food jungle. Neurotically, we yearn for somebody to rescue us from this jungle when we know, deep in our hearts, that we are that someone. The escape route is the path less traveled, but the trend is that most people follow each other into the jungle, no questions asked. Most of us get stuck in this jungle because we don't know how to escape. We haven't learned the Japanese method of politely bowing, and backing out with a smile. We settle to live our lives being trapped in the jungle because our impotent desire to escape has lost its momentum. Let's face it. More often than not we are consumers of fast, instant, and processed foods. For example, a meal today may still consist of potato spuds smothered in butter and gravy, a piece of steak surrounded with fat, a can of diet soda, and a generous slice of apple pie a-la-mode. Where is the fiber, the staple, our foundation? We know that today's high tech fat is a heavy hitter. Ask any failure. And haven't we failed in our diets at one time or another? The JFJ has only one type of serving, the typical high-fat, low-fiber meal. This type of diet causes us to be overweight and unhealthy within our body, mind, and soul. How can we survive this? We cannot survive this. We can only escape this fiber-forsaken junk food jungle. Fiber is an essential part of a healthful diet, and here is how it works. Because we lack the necessary enzymes to break down fiber, it passes through our gastro-intestinal tract as the untouchable. As it travels the distance of our digestive system it takes out our trash, thus leaving our bodies squeaky-clean. What is this nature machine? What is it made of?

Marcia Sheridan, R.N.

What is Fiber?

Fiber or roughage, as it's sometimes called is the part of plants that does the natural, waste-removal. In the old days, it was taken for granted. Today fiber is put upon a pedestal for its life-preserving properties. We also know that keeping the fiber in our foods is the best way to reap their benefits. As fiber passes through our digestive systems, it not only takes with it all the toxins and wastes that are present at the time, but it also allow water to be absorbed from the large intestines. Fiber has a beneficial cleansing effect on our digestive system that nothing can replace. It's like our immune system. The two types of fiber are soluble and insoluble. Soluble fiber dissolves in water while insoluble fiber does not. Insoluble fiber is most effective in preventing constipation. It's mostly found in bran, wheat, fruits, and vegetables. However, all fruits, vegetables, and whole grains contain different amounts of each type of fiber. Because our contemporary culture is the largest producers and consumer of processed foods, we must consciously reintroduce fiber into our diet to help counteract the complications of such foods. We can add fiber to our diets through smart decisions at the grocery store (choosing natural foods like potatoes instead of potato spuds or chips). It is best to avoid high-fat, low-fiber meals, but, if you do eat more fat than you care to admit, then add some fiber. By adding fiber (i.e., bran) to your diet you can lessen the build-up of fat and pressure in the gastro-intestinal (GI) tract. Increased pressure on the GI tract is associated with the development of colon cancer. Other associations are heart disease, hemorrhoids, varicose veins, high cholesterol, and diverticulitis. High-fat and high-cholesterol meals are by definition devoid of fiber. They contribute to the greatest difficulty in waste disposal. Is waste disposal important for good health? Is exhaling important in keeping us alive? Absolutely! Therefore we must talk a little on this uncomfortable topic. Although you may think nothing of it, a lack of fiber in our diet affects our health; it shows in our dependence on stool softeners, laxatives and the like. We cannot inhale without exhaling; we must get rid of the carbon dioxide in our lungs. Equally, it's important to get rid of waste from our digestive system in order to maintain a healthy balance.

Natural Fiber Supplements

Picture this ladies: a peachy looking peach-the beauty of it, the texture of it, the smell of it, and the taste of each juicy bite. Imagine one little, Georgia peach stimulating all five of our senses simultaneously. And, after all that pleasure up front, she takes our waste away as she makes her exit. Wouldn't you be willing to escape the JFJ for a beautiful angel like her? I did. I love it. If a peach doesn't interest you try an apple a day, but make sure you get your groove back before you hit the grave. Supplementing one's diet with an apple, a raw carrot (cooked carrots elevate blood sugar rapidly) or a small, green salad during your meal may do the trick. Having two spoonfuls of bran with a glass of water before bed will help to complete the healthful process of eating by helping your body to rid itself of waste.

Let me repeat, eliminating waste is as urgent and as necessary as eating when hungry. The wastes found in high-fat/cholesterol, low-fiber diets require prompt elimination. This prevents stagnation in the colon and re-absorption of toxins into the blood. Such speed decreases the risk for colon cancer, high cholesterol and overweight. A lack of fiber and water in our diet produces dryness and difficulty in waste disposal, what we call constipation. This condition causes excessive straining and holding of the breath during the elimination process. The holding of the breath increases one's blood pressure and lends itself to a possible heart attack. For some people, sometimes this extra pressure is exactly what brings on a heart attack. I have noticed that a significant number of medical patients have gone into cardiac arrest this way. Congestive heart failure can also be triggered in this case. So, ladies, a daily injection of fiber in our diet can instill calm and composure during the elimination process. Isn't that good news? We could actually enjoy the process as much as we enjoy eating. Why not, it's a normal part of life. We could get some good reading done without being stressed. For some of us, it may be the only break we get all day.

Marcia Sheridan, R.N.

Diverticulitis and Discomfort, Stress To The Last Drop

Another health risk related to straining when constipated is diverticulitis. Diverticulitis is more chronic and less fatal than CHF or a heart attack. It's a weakening of the walls of the intestines which causes herniation, pockets or out-pouching along these walls. Unwanted particles become lodged in these pockets (diverticuli), causing inflammation in the colon or other serious conditions such as cancer. Straining can also contribute to hemorrhoids , which are very painful. When the diet is low in fiber, there is less bulk for the intestine to work with. This slows the process of elimination of fat and refined foods which gives them more time to be completely absorbed and increase our weight. Hiatal hernia is another complication that can occur. This usually leads to indigestion, gas-pain and acid reflux. Lack of fiber can also causes serious constipation, which may require medical prescriptions.

Fiber And Our Hearts

Lack of fiber contributes to the development of heart and blood vessel diseases. As mentioned before, an absence of fiber in the presence of high-fat, high cholesterol meals allows complete absorption of the two into the blood stream. Over time they accumulate as plaque-build-up thus narrowing the lumen of the arteries supplying vital organs such as our brain and heart. With poor supply or no supply of blood to these organs we could experience a brain attack (stroke), or a heart attack. Who would think fiber could be so vital to our good health?

The Human digestive system And Fiber

The human animal has adapted to eating meats of all sorts. However, the human GI tract is very long, which is more suited for vegetarianism and diets that are much higher in fiber. Carnivores have a shorter and smoother bowel that is more suited for meat digestion. In a short system, meat is digested much faster. The shorter, more direct GI system handles fat and cholesterol very well. It also requires less fiber to move waste out of the intestines. This is why carnivores, such as lions, do not get colon cancer the way humans do. Our susceptibility to colon cancer most likely comes from our high-fat, high-cholesterol, and low-fiber diet. If we insist on eating meat, we should at least consume adequate amounts of fiber to aid in our digestion.

Fiber As A Friend

Although fiber is not a nutrient, its presence in the diet is vital for normal body functioning and the absorption of toxins. For example, fiber will slow down and decrease the absorption of sugar in the blood. This process helps tremendously in preventing blood sugar fluctuations and the onset of diabetes in some people. While fiber helps to bind some cholesterol and fat, thus preventing their absorption altogether, it also traps high levels of estrogen and rids the body of it via the feces. Without adequate fiber to trap estrogen, it will build up in the blood. It may affect organs that are sensitive to sex hormones and can lead to various types of cancer, in particular breast cancer. A high-fat diet of red meat, dairy products, and greasy fried foods contributes to the high levels of estrogen in young girls, which can cause premature puberty and female-related cancers. By simply adding fiber to a high-fat diet, you can make a positive difference instantly. It can cut a significant portion of that fat intake out of your system.

Fresh Fruits And Vegetables

This is the easiest and most simple way to live off the land. Picking fruits, and digging up roots is how I grew up. All fruits and vegetables provide lots of water and a kind of fiber called pectin. Pectin is largely found in raw carrots and apples and has been linked to lowering the levels of cholesterol in the blood. Fiber also traps and rids the body of bile salts. The body, in turn, draws cholesterol from the blood to replace the bile acids. This process helps to lower the cholesterol level in the blood. I have fruits every morning for breakfast. This is a nice way to warm up our bodies before we go into high gear. For those of us who cannot have a big heavy meal for breakfast, fruits are a fabulous alternative. Between my regular meals, I snack on fruits and vegetables to take the edge off my hunger. Fresh fruits can curb our cravings, cure our bad taste and cleanse our colon. When I'm in a rush, I grab a banana and an apple for breakfast in the car. This is usually enough to satisfy me until lunch. In between, I will have a glass of water at work. I always have a bottle of water for such times. Our dietary fiber should be obtained from many sources. Some excellent fruit choices are dried prunes, apples, pears, apricots, and nectarines. For lunch or dinner, I try to have a salad with a little lime or lemon juice. I find that salads kill my appetite in the afternoons (the cheating hours). Green, leafy vegetables are also rich in vitamin A, calcium, and iron. Spinach is one of my favorite green vegetables along with cucumbers. I sometimes make a drink with cucumbers during the summer for my bike rides. Its high water content is refreshing. One great advantage of the cucumber is that it requires more calories to be digested than it actually yields, and it is also high in water and fiber. It allows you to burn extra calories instead of adding calories to your meal. Before a competition, when I wanted to look lean, I'd consume large quantities of cucumbers, including the skin that contains most of the fiber. So keep in mind, ladies, we eat for good health, not just to please our palate and tickle our taste buds. For root vegetables, I like yams (sweet potatoes) and Irish potatoes. Sweet potatoes are great baked with apples and cinnamon. I steam my vegetables, and I'm very careful not to over cook them. I like the natural taste of vegetables when they're partially cooked. It's an acquired taste. Most of the nutrients in vegetables are destroyed when they're overcooked. They're usually ready when their color becomes brighter. Vegetables should be eaten at the bright color stage to capitalize on their vitamins and minerals.

Bran To The Rescue

When You Cheat, Being human, I sometimes cheat and have a cookie or two, or more. Sometimes it's a piece of chocolate. Other times, it's the entire chocolate bar. Ah, can you relate? Now that

I'm not a competitive athlete, I have more time for temptations, but less time to burn them off. My remedy for my occasional vulnerability is very simple. The wise action that I take is to have three teaspoons of bran with a glass of water. This works for me, and it can work for you also. Here is what happens, the fiber actually acts as a trap for the cookies and chocolate; thus, it decreases the rate of absorption, as well as the amount of sugars being absorbed. Most importantly, the bran prevents the rush I would have gotten from an elevated blood sugar. As a result it also prevents the desire to have more sugar. This is how we can nip the sugar roller coaster in the bud and regain some control. Not only does adding bran bring us great benefits of health it also helps to control our weight by increasing the transit time for food digestion while it decreases the caloric absorption. The food transit time is the amount of time it takes our digestive system to move food through the system. The bonus is that the added fiber helps with our daily cleansing, while it keeps us as regular as the clock on a daily basis. This is one clean "F" word in more ways than one. Fiber is indeed a friend we need.

How To Increase Fiber In Your Diet

Who are these fiber guys? They are good, old complex CHO. We can increase our fiber with complex CHO intake by making slow and small introductions of brown rice, fruits, vegetables (lots of vegetables), barley, beans of all shapes and sizes, oat bran, and whole grains in our diet. One of my favorites is good, old fashion oatmeal cereal with cinnamon and apples on top. Oatmeal is high in fiber and complex CHO. Its nutrients are kept intact after the rolling process, and it makes great muffins. **Good, old-fashioned oats is great.** Brown rice, whole wheat, beans, and soy pasta products are also natural ways to increase fiber in the diet, as well as complex CHO. For some of us, eating this way will be a turning point. But that's great, because it will allow us to enjoy life now, and later. With our complex CHO intake, we're increasing fiber in our diets as well as needed minerals and vitamins. For example, a raw carrot provides high fiber, complex CHO, and beta-carotene, which is great for our skin and our vision. It's considered an antioxidant, which helps to prevent cancers. Fiber helps to keep our blood thin by lowering cholesterol. Therefore it decreases periods of fatigue, irritability, tiredness, and emotional stress. We can all agree that we feel more stressed when we're tired and irritable. Who would think that fiber was so stress and pressure reducing, and life sustaining? I recommend taking two teaspoons of bran daily to add extra fiber to our diet if we're not as regular as we need to be. We should do this before or after a meal, because bran can prevent the absorption of zinc, iron, and calcium. You can sprinkle bran on your desserts for crunch and munch and a bunch of happy days. Increase your fiber intake gradually. Our intestines do need time to adjust to increased fiber. A sudden overdose of fiber may cause bloating, gas or intestinal irritations such as diarrhea, due to bacterial fermentation. Also, our intestinal bacteria need time to adjust to the breakdown process of fibers.

Wok Cooking

During the early part of my childhood, I often watched my Chinese relatives cook Chinese food in a wok. The smell was great, the taste was superb, and I would always look forward to Chinese New Year to enjoy some wonderful Chinese home cooking. I enjoy my dad's cooking even though I seldom see him. When he cooks, I ask him to use very little oil, which he does. I am now cooking the same way. Woks are great for stir-frying vegetables. You can lightly spray the wok to prevent sticking. With a hot wok, vegetables can be cooked very fast with very little fat. Just like shrimp, vegetables are also perfect for consumption when they are bright in color, but they're a lot more healthful than shrimp. Using the wok form of preparation, vegetables can be cooked just enough to retain all of their good flavor, vitamins, and minerals along with their fiber. We can also add bits of tofu, turkey, chicken, fish, or egg whites to complete our meal. These are ways to add protein to a high-fiber and complex CHO meal with very little fat. When you're unable to cook or you're on a trip, it's okay to have bran flakes or take fiber supplements to make do. But never lose track that our fiber should come naturally from the foods we eat and not mainly from over the counter laxatives. These are substances that were commonly prescribed for my medical patients, victims of complications related to lack of fiber in their diets. Here is another chance to escape.

The Fiber Water Connection

We need to let the fountain of youth flow freely through our veins and arteries. Along with increasing fiber, we need to increase our natural water intake. Fiber works well in the presence of water. Our bodies work well when water is present. We're made of eighty- percent water. Therefore, most of what we eat should be high in water. Our lymphatic system needs water to help flush the system and eliminate waste. Come to think of it, our system needs water to flush itself out the same way our toilet bowls do. Plain water, water-packed foods, and natural fruit juices are the best sources of water consumption. Water works well with soluble and insoluble fibers to cleanse, rejuvenate, and replenish some of the lost fluids. Water is the fluid of life. Without water, we would all die of dehydration. All bodily functions depend upon the presence of water. The body loses almost a gallon of water daily through respiration, perspiration, urination, and digestive waste. Fiber without water is not very helpful in aiding in the elimination process. Having the two together is paramount. Sufficient fiber and water every day can make your bowels move with effortless ease. Together they help to complete the connection between our intake and our output. They can give our heart a beating chance and make them a powerful force to fight the junk food jungle and promote health. In addition to weight loss by trapping some fats and sugars, and slowing their absorption, fiber can sometimes totally eliminate them from the body. A high-fiber diet always prevents blood sugar fluctuations by stabilizing the absorption of sugar as early as in the stomach, and it continues to do this as it moves down the line. Hopefully, I have convinced you that water and fiber together is the overall force for good health in our diet. Even if one were staunchly opposed to fibrous foods, I think the compelling benefits of a lower risk for heart disease, cancer, and obesity should persuade anyone to embrace fiber as a friend. A dear friend that will become more user-friendly with increased consumption. We can all relish the idea of fiber unlocking the door to a longer and more youthful life. On our self-care quest we can use fiber to help fight the battle of the bulge, the war against heart disease, and the soaring problem of high cholesterol that cuts across age groups. The battle against heart disease begins at birth. Water is the life force and fiber is the prolonging life source. Together they are the miracle couple of rejuvenation, youth, and vitality. We need to use whatever means we can to escape the junk food jungle. As we get older, water and fiber becomes more essential, because we're less active. Water and fiber is one delivery team that will never fail to deliver no matter what kind of weather we're having. Try them, and see how well they will work to get you through the JFJ. Even better, they will get the junk food jungle out of your system. Fiber and water is the force we need to join to get us through the long haul and a little closer to our desire to be fit, fun and free.

Chapter 6

Fad Diets, Diet Pills, Metabolism, and The Weight Loss Dilemma

Fad dieting is death and dying, **DIE -T-ING**. As you can see the first three letters spells death **(DIE)**. As soon as our bodies (as intelligent as they are) sense death they begin to fight back. The following are some real life issues we must look at under the microscope: .

The Connection Between Meals, Metabolism, and Weight Maintenance is to connect Intellectual Knowledge and Spiritual Wisdom to our Physical Practices.

- The Muscle Metabolism Connection
- The Effects Of A Low Caloric Diet On Our Bodies
- Commercial Weight Loss Programs
- The Connection Between Women on the Pill Who Smoke
- Caffeine
- GERD: Gastro-Esophageal Reflux Disease
- Diet Pills
- Beware Of Saboteurs, Don't Surrender Leadership To Them
- Lord Over Your Own Life

At some point in our lives most of us will go on a weight-reducing diet. The number of diets available is dazzling and mind-boggling, because, over the long haul, we know they don't work. We diet for many reasons: we want to lose weight after having a baby, we want to be attractive again, or perhaps for personal health and well being. Whatever our motivation is, we want to lose weight and look great, but, ironically, after the diet we sometimes look more overweight and feel worse than ever. Why do we gain more weight after the diet? When we first begin to lose weight, we will lose water. We can lose over ten pounds of water in a week or less. This is the success of most diets that promise rapid weight loss in a week or two. This could mean rapid death also. Since our bodies are 80% water, we should not be losing water and mistaking it for genuine weight loss. Our body will replace the water one way or another as soon as possible. This is exactly why such weight loss attempts is always short lived. Likewise, on a prolonged low-calorie diet, we program our bodies to function on fewer calories than before. This lowers our set point for food metabolism. Initially, we will lose some weight, but our bodies quickly adapt to function on fewer calories. The scale will show a loss in weight, but it does not tell us that the weight we have just lost was only water along with our precious muscles. The body stores fat when blood sugar falls due to inadequate intake of needed complex CHO calories. The body reacts as though there were a famine going on. It protects its fat storage by lowering our basal metabolic rate (BMR), the rate at which the body burns calories. This fall in BMR causes our body to burn fewer calories. It will hold onto the fat we already have and will also quickly convert what we eat into fat. What our bodies do on a low-calorie diet is to break down our precious muscles for its energy source. This leaves our muscles weaker, smaller, and flabbier, and we're left with poor physical fitness. On a low-calorie diet, we tend to become frustrated and irritable quickly. That is because our blood sugar level is below normal. A prolonged low blood sugar will keep us feeling hungry all the time. Eventually the drive to eat over-powers our will to lose weight. Our bodies will be screaming for some real food almost 24 hours a day. Most people go off this diet before they're able to reach their ideal weight. If our willpower is strong enough to take us to our goal weight, as soon as we discontinue the diet and begin to have our regular meals, our body will even more rapidly store the excess food as fat! We will not burn it off, because our metabolism will have been lowered. This is another defensive and protective mechanism used by the body to combat the sense of starvation. We're now physically weaker and more vulnerable both spiritually and emotionally than we were before we went on our low-calorie diet. Our weight baseline is elevated (meaning the body is set to function at a higher weight). It is now able to maintain this extra weight on fewer calories. Therefore, even if we maintain our intake we will inevitably store more fat. Our low-calorie diet would have done great harm to our BMS. Unfortunately we will have bought into wasted time, energy and money. It's what Jamaicans call buying a puss in a bag. The point is these diets serve only to separate us from our money, not our fat. We all know that most people are fatter and heavier after the diet. By now, we must realize that quick fixes only work for flat tires. Proper weight loss requires more, because we're asking for more. A basic foundational change in lifestyle is what we need, and this requires knowledge, discipline and persistence working harmoniously to complete our connection to purpose.

The Muscle Metabolism-Connection

Muscles are the essential physical tools necessary to exercise, RAISE OUR METABOLISM, and burn our unwanted fat. Without muscles, our hands are tied and our fat cravings can run rampant. The more fat cells we have, the more we're drawn to fatty foods. While on a low calorie diet, we could have lost twenty percent of our muscle mass as weight loss while thinking we have lost fat. This will give us less ammunition to work with in trying to lose weight the proper way in the future. The scale can be misleading. As long as we see weight loss, we feel good. But the scale is not always the best judge. A muscle to fat ratio test, or our reflection in a mirror, is better. This allows us to see our bodies and to experience our feelings towards our reflection in the mirror. When we're honest, we can see we do not look or feel any better. In fact, we may be genuinely unhappy and broken on the inside. If we're honest we won't try to lie to the woman in the mirror, we will seek wisdom and a genuine approach to weight loss. Women need to realize the value of muscles. Muscle loss makes it difficult to carry out the activities of daily living without experiencing fatigue, irritability, and the urge to eat fast sugar for energy. Having lost muscle mass, we can have a flabby appearance, excess skin, stretch marks, or looseness between our skin and bones. No one wants to flab, sag, or waddle like a duck. Can women develop muscles that say fit, fun, and feminine on a starvation diet? No. A well-toned muscular physique will always have a tighter and a more youthful appearance, but in order to develop this, we must eat wisely and exercise regularly.

Marcia Sheridan, R.N.

The Side Effects of a Low Calorie Diet on our Bodies

Some of the adverse effects of a low calorie diet that causes or contributes to common diseases in American women today are:
1) Fatigue
2) Dizziness
3) Nervousness
4) Headache
5) Agitation
6) Listlessness
7) Irritability
8) Depression
9) Inability to concentrate
10) High blood pressure.
11) PMS
12) Mental Stress Overload

In response to all of these side effects, our body experiences tremendous spiritual, emotional, and physical stress, the "fight or flight" syndrome. Humans and other animals will experience the fight or flight syndrome when confronted with real or imagined danger. Our programmed, unconscious, automatic response, is to escape such dangers instantly. But, in our contemporary concrete jungle, we've anesthetized our feelings and allowed our stress to build into mountains we're unable to climb. When faced with stress real or imagined our body will secrete nor-epinephrine (adrenaline) into the blood, speed up our heart rate, constrict our blood vessels, and elevate our blood pressure. This is the mechanics of the fight or flight response. It's nature's way of preparing us to defend our position. This process happens in seconds, and it happens weather the stress is real or not, because our unconscious does not distinguish real from imagined dangers. This fight or flight response, is what people mean when they say, "my adrenaline was pumping." We cannot afford to let ourselves sit and marinate in the juices of contemporary stress. Such stress is an unnecessary self-induced drain of our energy, it disconnects us from genuine joy. When we experience any of the side effects of a low-calorie diet, our body goes through the fight or flight syndrome, as if the diet was a threat. Indeed it is, our body is wiser than we are. Our body will secrete adrenaline (nor-epinephrine) and elevate our heart rate and blood pressure. These symptoms inflict constant physical and emotional stress on our body. These stresses contribute to our experience of headaches, light-headedness or irritability. Headaches and irritability almost always create grouchiness. No one wants to be a grouch or to be around one. This is how closely connected our diet, blood pressure, and mood swings are. The energy we get from our adrenaline rush is not a good source of energy. To function on this source of energy puts great stress on all the systems of the body. Adrenaline energy should be used only in rare cases of emergency. Most women once thought that a low-calorie diet was a good way to lose weight, not realizing how adversely they affect our hearts, and minds. Imagine the degree of stress on our hearts in this constant state of fight or flight. Over the years, this kind of stress on our body will ruin our health, and kill our desire for good health. A stressed out burned out body will produce a rebellious personality. One that has lost the connection from its spiritual energy and purpose. Losing control means allowing stress to abuse our bodies physically and emotionally. Is it any wonder that the leading health problems and cause of death are heart attacks, brain attacks (strokes) and cancer, especially in women?

Commercial Weight Loss Programs

I think it's important to take a look at our diets and make the appropriate changes. I am not interested in being in the weight loss business, however. Most weight loss programs are just too much ado about nothing. My feeling is that a lot of the weight-loss programs that I know about have been in the business for years. People have been going on and off such programs for years. Unfortunately, they've been gaining more weight after each program. That is because weight loss programs can't give us a program that lasts forever. If they did, the program's success would put them right out of business. People like to spread good news. They would be glad to tell you how it works for free. The only thing that works for us is our own commitment to ourselves. This "burst bubble syndrome" is true for most programs. They are not miracles, they may help us to get started, but, at some point, we have to take over and do it ourselves. The best way to do this is to first make a definite decision to change our lifestyle. Spiritual food is also necessary to maintain harmony and balance within our body. We must fertilize the soil of our spirit with universal wisdom in order to evolve into complete health. Our soul's divinity deserves to be discovered and loved because it is a large part of who we are. We must also cultivate positive thoughts as food for our minds. Second, we must educate ourselves. Reading lots of articles and books on spirituality, emotional health and lifestyle improvements. Such knowledge in action can bring great results. We can no longer ignore the inner elements of our being. If we're to completely connect to our entire being, then it is wise to nurture and nourish our mind and spirit along with our body. Back to the diet dilemma. Rigid diet programs are not for us anymore. We have completed our connection to a healthy lifestyle at least in our minds and spirits. But don't worry we'll be healthy in body soon, because where ever our spirits lead our bodies will follow naturally. Allow me to share with you my heart-felt emotion about a very special soul. I won't say her name, but I know you know who she is, if you don't now, you will in time. We've watched one of America's most famous personality connect completely to body, mind and spirit. I now feel her connection to my spirit, just as my spirit is now connected to yours. This invisible force towards health body, mind and spirit is like a global chain reaction. Once we become conscious of our authentic heart's desire to be completely healthy our spirits are drawn towards complete connection to each other. OK. This lady told us on national TV that she could not live on the program that helped her to lose 68 pounds years ago. That it was very unhealthy for her physically, mentally and spiritually. Her entire being rebelled on that straight-jacket, draining and deadly diet. We watched her regain the weight and suffered the consequences. But she was persistent and wise enough to connect to the source of her inner spiritual strength. Today she is completely connected individually and collectively with our spirits. Together as women we can completely connect a spiritual force that will make us healthy and whole. Yes, and without commercial diet programs. The genuine program that we all need to stay the course of health and fitness is the program of collective global spiritual exchange of energy. In that we desire good health for all people not just ourselves. We must then send this desired intention to the universal spirit, our source of creation to be connected as one spiritual force. As a unified force we can collectively enjoy our individual desires because our individual inner strength will come from ever living, ever loving, universal Jah love. This is a belief about the future of our health that I share deeply. I don't believe that our authentic and lasting health will come from weight loss programs, but from our desire to accept, love and help each other as we are. It will definitely be a divine deliverance, not a monetary program.

I am not selling any weight loss programs, vitamins, foods, or gym equipments. My motivation is to persuade, galvanize, spiritualize, and make you aware of health risks and ways that we all can help to prevent illnesses. I'm interested in moving in a new direction. One we have not taken before; it's a global, spiritual, and unified approach towards total health and fitness for all people. I am an R.N., and I give great injections. In this book my hope is to inject you with spiritual energy and theoretical knowledge chose a new path away from the junk food jungle and towards a healthy lifestyle BMS. Follow your path of spiritual connection and inspiration within this deep ocean of chaos. You'll be able to face and fix any of your diet dilemmas without the aid of any commercial weight loss nightmares.

The Connection Between Women On The Pill Who Smoke

Smoking is not recommended ever as an appetite suppressant; it is even more dangerous for women on the pill. It puts them at high risk for heart disease; and if they should get pregnant they risk miscarriages and lower-birth weight babies. Their babies are also prone to sudden death. Breast-feeding mothers increase the incidence of passing nicotine to their babies through their breast milk. I can help women who are over-weight, but I can't help women or babies with cancer. Ladies, we need you to be healthy, smoke free and cancer free. You can always work wonders with weight, but not cancer. I've been talking about healthy diets throughout this book. It's prudent to eat healthful foods. Therefore I believe it would be destructive to have a cigarette right after a healthful meal. Don't give up. Ladies we're all in this struggle together.

Caffeine

The consumption of coffee is very similar to cigarette smoking. The active ingredient is caffeine, it artificially increase our basal metabolic rate (BMR). This allows us to burn more calories. However this is not a healthful way to raise our metabolism, or to lose weight. Coffee is a two-edged sword, while it increases the BMR it also triggers the release of insulin into the blood. This in turn lowers our blood sugar, and triggers a hunger response. While one, or two, cups a day is okay, we should remember that we could become addicted to the caffeine jolt. Also, if you're one to put a lot of cream in your coffee, you could end up gaining far more weight than you expect because cream is mostly fat. We get incredible hips. Coffee also acts as a diuretic and causes the body to lose necessary water. This can lead to dehydration, or loss of necessary vitamins, electrolytes, and minerals via the urine. This could be mistaken for significant weight loss.

Gastro Esophageal Reflux Disease (GERD)

Excess coffee also contributes to GERD, gastro- esophageal-reflux- disease, this is when we experience heartburn in our stomach, or in our throat because the gastric juices in the stomach are rebounding. Adding more cream is not helpful, it's just adding more incredible, spreadable flab to our hips. Enjoy your coffee, but please keep it to two cups a day; I too enjoy a cup here and there.

Diet Pills

Appetite Suppressants: works by influencing the shut-off, of our appetite center. This decreases our appetite. This like all the other drugs can be harmful because it's unnatural. Most suppressants do not affect appetite. Instead, they create an artificial, drug-induced increase in our basal metabolic rate(BMR), and arrest our system into a flight or fight condition all day long. Appetite suppressants can cause rapid heartbeat, palpitations, and hallucinations and, in some cases, they can be fatal. Depending on how low our caloric intake our body will function by breaking down our muscles for energy. We can lose up to one pound of muscle for every pound of fat we lose. On the scale, we may be lighter; however, in reality, we will be flabbier and will have a higher percentage of body fat in comparison to our muscle mass. Again, appetite suppressants are just like nicotine and coffee in that they also artificially stimulate our BMR, and trigger the fight or flight syndrome. Diet aids are just another avenue that will take us to the never-never-land of self-destruction, poor health, and stress. Remember our mantra we're into good health for the long haul, and if it's going to happen, it's up to "US".

Beware of Saboteurs, Don't Surrender Leadership to Them, Lord Over Your Own Life

Most importantly, we should never give away our power. We have the power to know and decide what's best for us. Most of these bad habits were developed during the teen years for some of us, at a time when we were not aware of our saboteurs. We were essentially seduced mentally while we believed they were helping us. Saboteurs are not really thinking about us. They're thinking about how much money they can take from us. They sell empty promises and turn us into helpless addicts over the long haul. Obviously we're turning the tables on them by educating ourselves. Knowing the benefits of a healthful life-style makes it easier to follow. Looking younger after one stops smoking is an incentive. Feeling healthier and trimmer on healthful, low-fat, natural food is rewarding and is worth the struggle. Watching our children grow up healthy and being able to enjoy life with them are worthwhile reasons to live healthfully. Taking total charge of our health is what women are about for the twenty-first century. We want to uncover and

Marcia Sheridan, R.N.

discover a new and better way of life. When we reach the point of understanding that we will no longer need crutches, and we're determined not to quit; then, and only then, are we guaranteed that we will succeed. When our need to succeed is a blazing fire, we will be unstoppable. We will escape the junk food jungle and find a place of permanent peace within and without. Spirituality and love for self and others is our passport to a heaven of health and happiness. We will disconnect from the destructive jungle of foods and fears; as we ascend into the new millenium, a new age of enlightenment, spirituality, global cultural consciousness and a time to experience our connection completely.

Chapter 7

Part l
Daily Dietary Devotions To Launch Women Into Lasting Health; Away From Obesity, Heart Disease, And Breast Cancer

- Eating guidelines
- Regular Meals
- Size Vs Intervals
- Variety In Our Diet
- Avoid Eating Late
- The Connection Between Advanced Plans and Preparation of Meals
- Seek Support
- Being Role Models For Ourselves
- What's The Connection Between Kids Diet and Adult Diet?
- How To Escape The Hunk Food Jungle of Fast Food, Fast Fat and Snack Attacks
- Cut The Grease And The Guilt, Avoid High Fat Heavy Hitters
- Dining Out Low Fat
- Holiday Dining
- Why Can't I Just Pig Out On Meats For The Holiday?
- How Can We Replace Fat?

How can we hijack our diets into the right zone? In order to become Ms. Natural America, I had to drastically change my eating style. I'd like to share with you some of the tips I know. Because I changed my eating style, I have been able to maintain my weight for sixteen years. Losing weight improperly is easy compared to becoming healthy and fit. We need to share some realistic goals for losing weight and keeping it off permanently. A ship without a rudder will move in any direction. Here are some long-term general rules that have allowed me to lose fat and keep fit for the past fifteen years. You too can benefit from these eating guidelines:

Eating Guidelines

(1) Eat **regular meals** three to five times a day as hunger dictates, preferably at the same times.

(2) Eat **small meals** (portions).

(3) Keep **variety** in your diet.

(4) Plan to eat **before 6:30 p.m.**

(5) Plan and **prepare your own** meals (fruit drinks, tossed salads, and fruit salads for in-between meals as hunger-pacifiers).

(6) Avoid **fast foods** and high-fat foods.

(7) Exercise at least three times per week, even when you don't feel like exercising. If you do it, it will work. A study done in Norway showed that even four hours of exercise per week will decrease a woman's chance for breast cancer and lower her fat ratio. Moderate exercise decreases our risk 25%, while it keeps us in better shape physically and emotionally. This study was done in the early nineties, but it still holds true today.

(8) Try to get at least seven to **eight hours of sleep** at night.

(9) When eating out, **check the menu carefully**. Ask the waiter for recommendation of dishes that are low- fat or non-fat. (Ask for all sauces, dressings, and butter to be served on the side).

(10) Refrigerate canned soups to harden any fat, then **ladle off the fat. This trick can turn any soup fat free**.

(11) It's not easy to say **" no"** to foods that will sabotage your goals because they're just like drugs. Once you start you could get hooked. Every time we eat inappropriately we deepen the roots of harmful habits. We must instead keep picturing and visualizing the new connection we want to make. Equally we must link pleasure to the power of choice.

(12) What do you do when those junk food urges creep up to disconnect you from your goal? First thing to do is to have a glass of water, and **wait five minutes**. If you do this, your urge will subside. Practice and patience are not just a virtues here;

they are the keys to complete our connection to *the good life*.

Regular Meals

Regular meals are our bodyguard against those sweet snack attacks. Our wise body will prepare itself for digestion at regularly scheduled meal times. Because it needs a steady source of energy in the blood. When we delay or miss meals our blood sugar falls. Our brain does not get the constant energy source it requires to keep us alert. This low blood sugar level causes us to feel fatigue, weak, tired and irritabile. Skipping meals is how we set ourselves up for self-sabotage and bad eating habits. Skipping meals and lowering our blood sugar puts us out of control of our intake, and make us vulnerable to sugar cravings. Anything sweet becomes our sweet heart. But it's not a case of sweets for the sweet; it's sweets for the "BEAST". For example, we may begin to have a cup of coffee and then find ourselves having donuts, cookies, cake, or a candy bar.

I cannot emphasize enough, the importance of planning ahead and having regular meals. Planing our meals and exercise routines are weapons against temptation. Regular meals take care of our vulnerability to sweets by supplying a steady source of energy to our brain. This is where your complex CHO will play their best game in helping you win against the temptations of a low blood sugar. Sporadic eating will not just affect you physiologically. It can also ruin your psychology of discipline. Please, don't skip breakfast. Plan ahead to prevent failure. Failure is not a good place to be, don't go there.

Size Vs Interval

I have found that whenever I wait too long to eat, my appetite will be so great that I will eat a much larger portion. This behavior is not unique to me. In fact it's not unique to humans. Studies on the eating style of laboratory animals have confirmed the same behavior. They have found that the size of a meal was directly connected to the interval between each meal. A longer interval meant a larger meal. Larger meals cause the stomach and intestines to expand. Food was absorbed forty percent faster causing weight gain, calorie-for-calorie, as compared to eating at regular scheduled intervals.

I have personally experienced all of those findings. I believe this to be true for all of us. When our stomachs are constantly stretched, they will require more food to experience a sense of fullness. This will cause us to eat more and more at each meal. This will keep expanding our stomach and the cycle will continue until we reduce our portion sizes. One way to do this is to use smaller plates instead of large plates. They require less food to fill up and a full plate will trick our eyes into satisfaction. We eat with our eyes as much as with our mouths. We must train our eyes along with our brain to consume less and less at each meal until our intake is in harmony with our needs. This way we eat for success as much as we dress for success. Today we all want success. We can first claim it in our diets by controlling what, and how much we pack into our plates. That's being pro-active and taking charge.

Variety in Our Diets

It is good practice to vary our diets. It's quite easy to have different foods for each meal. Once a week or so, it's okay to have leftovers. Just don't eat the same foods three or four times in a row. One of my single girlfriends would make a large meal on weekends, to feed her for the entire week. She lit candles and prayed for a date to rescue her from her own cooking, and the boredom of having the same thing all week. Variation in the diet will prevent boredom. It will allow us to meet all our nutritional requirements. Variation also prevents one from feeling punished, or deprived. It helps prevent food allergies. Eating the same foods frequently can cause food allergies. Usually the allergic symptoms are so subtle that we may not connect them with our diets.

Avoid Eating Late

Once in a while, we may be able to get away with eating late. However, it's not a good practice. Foods eaten later in the day, or right before bed, cannot be burned completely because the body's metabolism slows down as the day progresses and it slows way down during sleep. Food eaten later in the day will most likely be stored as fat. My body fat significantly decreased within weeks after learning this fact. Initially, when I first started working out late at night, I went home looking forward to a big meal at 10:00 p.m. right before I went to sleep. I learned it wasn't okay just because I was working out every day. In fact, eating late at night was sabotaging my hard work. I realized my body fat was not reducing as much as it should have been. I can remember I would even wake up in the middle of the night and have a snack. Although I wasn't getting any fatter (because I was active) I wasn't losing fat as fast as I should have. One good thing that was in my favor was that I burned off most of my fat while I slept. Do you know why? Well, when you have a lot of muscles that are constantly rebuilding and repairing, you will burn more energy even at rest, than someone who doesn't exercise. This happens even while we sleep. Suffice it to say that if you're not active at all and you do eat late in the evenings (or at night), you can expect to gain even more weight than if you ate earlier. We need to eat at a decent hour in the evenings, at least three to four hours before we go to sleep.

The Connection Between Advance Plans And Preparation Of Meals

Prepare meals in advance and take them with you. This connection can curb the beast in long before it ever gets out bounds. My minister Robert Schuller Jr. once said: "What would you attempt to do if you knew you could not fail?" I promise you, if you approach this program of self-preservation with planning and preparation and a connection to your inner source of strength, you will not fail. Planned meals helps to avoid impulsive actions. The big benefits of bringing lunch to work: 1). When friends at work say, "Let's do lunch today," you can say I'd love to but I have my homemade lunch. 2). It is also a great time to quiet our mind, connect with our spirit, don't think about food so much and escape from stress. 3). We can use this time to find a quiet place to relax, and listen to our favorite music. I usually go into my office where I can *put my feet up, rejuvenate, meditate, visualize and pray for my heart's desires.* It's a time I've made to consume my mental and spiritual diet as well as my lunch. It's a ritual I observe even at home. At home I add a cup of tea to the ritual and consider it my, "Daily Mental-Mini-Vacation short and sweet." In cases however, when we do join our friends we can bring a bottle of water; and while they eat we can have a drink, hydrate our body while we visit and catching up with each other. One of my wisest and most successful moves was taking my non-fat lunch to work every day. Bringing lunch allowed me a longer break. I was finished eating before any one got out of the lunch line which took over thirty minutes sometimes. Eating before everyone else gave me more time to chew and enjoy my lunch and to resist temptations. Because I was already full I could honestly **say no thank you** and mean it from my heart. That's a powerful feeling, a feeling of self-control. I had more time to read my books and escape mentally. Sometimes I even went for a walk to boost up my energy level for the afternoon lag time, while I exercise and burn some calories. An ounce of planing in action is better than a pound of fat sitting down! Consistent smart plans made and followed, always deliver big benefits while it keep us on purpose for the long haul.

Seek Support

Whenever we're observing a healthful diet, it is wise to encourage support by sharing our plans and purpose with friends. This forces us to carry them out. Keeping our newly informed health plan a secret could mean that we we're not very serious or committed to our goals. It could also be that we don't have enough confidence in ourselves our ability and our ability to stick to our goals. When we tell people of our plans we also tell ourselves that we mean business. This is one way to send a serious message to our consciousness. It also builds character and conviction. It's a way to unleash the inner strength that is dying to support our authentic heart's desire. Finally we must honor the promises we make to ourselves in order to be healthy within and without. Don't let the fear of failure rob you of your birthright. You deserve a healthy life. Remember that fear is not an iron curtain. We can walk through it. We can be the leaner, healthier women we want to be. Improving our health and fitness is a big advantage—plus we'll find that as our weight decreases, our self-esteem and spirits will increase. Isn't that a great thing to strive for? My feeling is that when we share our goals with friends, we earn their support. Our own self-respect will increase as well. Friends will know not to offer or tempt us with undesirable foods. If people disrespect your purpose they're not friends. They should be avoided, if it's not possible on the job, then certainly in our personal lives. The healthful lifestyle that I cherish is applicable to anyone and is available to everyone.

Being Role Models for Ourselves

When we stand firm to our purpose no one can stand in our way. We will be victorious if we truly and deeply desire to be. As you can see, I do not advocate dieting or specific portions of foods. I believe that our body, our mind and our spirit are wise and intelligent, and will tell us when to stop eating. All we need to do is to listen with our hearts. I am specifically telling you what foods to avoid and what foods to embrace and why. We need not suffer from lack of knowledge. My intention in this book is to help educate, enlighten, and encourage you to help yourselves to healthier lifestyle. At this moment my heart felt desire is to seduce you into finding your own way and your connection to good nutrition, exercise and lasting health. In my heart I believe that this intention is a spiritual one, and is part of my purpose on this planet. My family and I now enjoy great health and fitness in our new lifestyle. However I'm aware that most people do not enjoy good health for various reasons. Therefore I feel lead to include you, my universal spiritual family in sharing in this complete connection to health and harmony. If you're a mother your family will benefit from your improved lifestyle. You can explain, practice, and tell them; but being an example is the best way to teach. Children as well as adults do what they see more than what they are told. My experience with my husband and my son has convinced me. I started my new, healthful lifestyle after my son's birth. He grew up watching me live a healthy lifestyle, which made it a completely natural, connection for him. He knows the connection between diet and health. He calls junk foods **killer foods**, as I told him. He points out TV commercials, saying, "Mom, look at all those killer foods." I am very relieved that I gave my son the gift of a health lifestyle. I feel it's my best gift to him and to the kids I hope he will have some day. I desire to connect to my loved ones the importance of health and fitness, long after I'm gone. The gift of health is a great connection for all of us to leave behind. Eric is a serious athlete who was awarded MVP (Most Valuable Player) on his baseball team, he has a black belt in tae- kwon- do, and he has now made the ALL-STAR team in baseball four years in a row. Eric aspires to be a pro-base ball player some day. He has a plan and purpose that keeps him connected. He is my hero and my role model as much as I am his. Today he is an inspiration to me; he helps me to keep in shape. I won't let him down by failing. We now eat and work out together with the same purpose at heart.

What's the Connection Between Kids Diet And Adult Diet?

A child or a teenager can eat the same type of foods that adults do. It should be in different portions, depending on the child. Kids should not be put on calorie-restrictive diets. Their growing bodies need a wholesome diet. Parents can improve their dietary consumption to accommodate their kid(s). A healthy lifestyle is better maintained when the entire family is involved. The biggest difficulty is making the children go without sweets. Small portions are okay especially around Halloween. Just have them drink lots of water. Kids tend to be much better at burning off sugar than are adults.

How to Escape The JFJ Of Fast Foods, Fast Fats And Snack Attacks

Fast foods are too fast to do any good but slow enough to do a lot of damage to our hips, hearts, and health. Fast foods are low in water content as well as fiber. The preparation of fast foods is unhealthy. Take french fries, for example. They are deep fried in saturated fats. They are sprinkled with excess salt, and more salt is added when ketchup is added. If there is any nutrient present, it's not worth the fat, cholesterol, or heart burn. How can we find the oasis deep in the desert of the junk food jungle? We find a salad bar, and chew on that as a drink. A salad bar may be the best way for us to survive in a fast food restaurant, providing we skip the regular high-fat salad dressing. We can substitute lemon juice, or a fat-free dressing. We're wise to skip the cheese, bacon bits, and the pasta that is swimming in oil. Even if it's olive oil (it's still fattening), it might not be as harmful to our heart, but it is a heavy hitter on our hips. Sometimes vegetable soups or grilled chicken that are low in fat are available. Although fast food restaurants are not where you should be dining, if you do get cornered in one, you may still come out as sturdy as Gibraltar, never having faltered. A good diet of salads, soups, baked potatoes, and grilled chicken will do. Whenever you feel doomed to disaster in the JFJ drink a glass of water very slowly. It will wash away our urges and erase the guilt that would follow. In the end we will feel gratitude, not grief.

Cut the Grease and the Guilt?
Avoid High Fat Heavy Hitters

High-fat foods are usually fast foods. Or is it that fast foods are usually high-fat foods? Twenty one million Americans on a daily basis consume high-fat fries. They consume seven billion pounds per year; and here is the clincher, each serving is over "20" big grams of fat. The greasy hamburger, double cheeseburger, greasy spare ribs, and various deep-fried chickens are examples of high-fat foods. As speaker for the American Heart Association I'm aware that lower income urban areas are the major consumers of fast foods in America in proportion to the rest of the population. They are also the ones to suffer high blood pressure and heart disease at an earlier age. They also die younger than mainstream America. Some African Americans are vulnerable to the high fat and high salt content in fast foods. They seem to have a higher incident of diabetes, and high blood pressure. The Latin American community is also hit hard by these two health hurricanes. However we're all potential candidates for such health risks. The JFJ is one world like it or not. It does not care who we are, it spells hell for us in more ways than one when we disconnect from the inner source of our strength.

Dining Out Low Fat

It is time to skip the gravy train and get on board the low fat lifestyle for the new millenium. First of all, pick restaurants with reasonable menus. Even in a restaurant we need to keep our focus, our purpose, and our commitment to healthy living. Dining out is not an escape from reality or the junk food jungle. It should not become a feeding frenzy or a culinary overdose. However it can be a delightful, healthful, and spiritual experience. The rules of eating low-fat still apply in a restaurant. We may not have total control as we would at home; however, good judgment and moderation is the key. Our ultimate success is dependent on our personal practices, not our social posturing. After all, no one else can keep track and keep control over what we put into our mouths. We can order plain for the main course and then add some of our own style to it. We can order a plain baked potato, plain boiled rice, or a plain salad, and take the trimmings on the side. Order baked, broiled, or grilled main courses instead of fried foods. Be the first one to order to resist the temptation or pressure to go overboard. Eat half of the serving and bring a doggie bag home. We can also split a main course with someone to save money and fat calories. Order dishes with marinara sauce. Skip the cream sauces. Don't forget to cleanse before a meal with a glass of water, and to flush at the end of the meal the same way. This is one way to get enough water intake while keeping our intake smaller. It is not impossible to dine out and enjoy a nice meal. Remember we eat for nourishment first and foremost, the principle of pleasure is mostly a mind game. We can enjoy low fat as an acquired taste. It will take some of us more time to acquire. However, good company, a nice atmosphere, and great service adds to the pleasure and the enjoyment of our meal. When ordering dairy, opt for non-fat dairy foods. This will reduce fat intake, cholesterol, and potential allergies. People develop allergies to dairy products very readily. Also, as we get older, some people have difficulty digesting dairy products, especially milk. Using the enzyme lactase will help in digesting milk and spare us the embarrassing flatulence (gas). We might think of dairy products as high protein foods. However, they are just as high in fat, if they're not the low- or non-fat types.

Holiday Dining

What should you do when dining out during the holidays? On holidays such as Thanksgiving, pick the white meat of the turkey and avoid the dark high/fat parts. Have less gravy and eat smaller portions, including dessert. Have a glass of water before the meal, and keep a glass on hand for the conclusion of your meal. Have a salad before you go to dinner if it will help you to maintain control. Empowerment here requires spiritual *psycho-physical* (mind-body) control over those holiday *hip-hop, high fat heavy hitters*. I know what a challenge such control can be, especially in the meat and gravy department. Ooh boy I can see it, I can smell it and I can taste it in my mind; I have been there and done that. In fact many times I too am tempted from time to time.

However, allow me to burst your holiday bubble by giving you a few facts. Our body will react to saturated fats no matter what holiday we're celebrating. Consuming less meat as we get older is a wise and prudent practice. It will help the most to prevent rapid premature aging.

Why Can't I Just Pig Out On Meats For The Holidays?

Well the truth is, you can. The problem is, there are too many holidays, too much food, and the food is usually decadent. As I have emphasized throughout this book, high-fat foods such as animal products put us at great risk for such ailments as breast and colon cancer and heart disease. Heart disease is connected to saturated animal fat, which is connected to plaque build up in our blood vessels, which is connected to a poor supply of nutrient rich blood to our heart. This causes our heart to be over worked and under paid. It is also the reason for premature wrinkling and aging of our skin, loss of youth and premature death. Now aren't you more willing to eat less meats on holidays? Besides in addition to child bearing and child rearing, today's women are being exposed to second hand smoke. Some of us drink and smoke, not just on holidays. We're candidates for heart disease and premature aging now, more than ever. Our bodies don't care what occasions we chose to celebrate, where we are, or who prepared the meal. We will get the same results for the same actions; our body cannot be tricked period.

How Can We Replace Fat?

Why do I spend so much time talking about "fat?" Reducing our fat intake as much as possible is the one most important thing we can do to lose weight and gain health. Keeping fat out of our diet is important to keep fat off of our bodies. The more body fat one has, the less we want to exercise. Obese individuals experience more sluggishness and are therefore more sedentary. This leads to more fat storage and even less desire to exercise. Excess fat in our diet is a temptation for our fat storing tendencies. The body loves to store fat so don't give it any. With a higher percentage of body fat, we burn less fat. We need to remember to weave exercise and complex CHO into our lives while we're removing the fat. They help us to control our impulsive eating by increasing the serotonin level in our brain. They also give us lots of energy to exercise and burn fat. We can eat in peace knowing that complex CHO will not make us fatter and is not associated with heart disease. Keep in mind that a little fat can be flavorful, but too much is a foe. Moderation is the armor of protection we wear to fight fat and cholesterol. This is a fight to the finish that we must win; but it's not the size of the woman that matters, it's the size of the fight inside the woman that does. Join with me and complete the connection we have made to authentic health and happiness for the long haul..

Chapter 7

Part ll
The Direct Connection Between Women's Diet And The Diseases They Develop Such As: Obesity, Heart Disease, Breast Cancer And Other Diseases In Women

- High Cholesterol
- Diet and Lifestyle
- Lack of Exercise
- Obesity
- The Connection Between Pregnancy and: Diet, Fitness, And Our Hearts
- The Connection Between Fat and Breast Cancer
- Emtional Stress

It is only fair for me to tie it all together for you now. I have been talking about heart disease, the junk food jungle, stress, exercise, diets, spirituality, mind and body and how they're all interconnected. We've also talked about acquiring strength from our inner source, and completing the connection to our purpose. But I haven't really isolated the issues of how to use what we have learnt so far to prevent, reverse, or control some of the related diseases women develop. So let me talk about how you can invest your time, energy and money in the business of *" your health and disease prevention incorporated"*.

Heart disease, obesity, and cancers are some of the most common preventable diseases women battle today. They are deeply connected to our diet, our lifestyle, and our stress level. The good news is that we can prevent or control them with diet and lifestyle modifications. In observing the principles we have just discussed in chapter seven part one we can make every effort to prevent these diseases. I think it's important to take a close look at some of these conditions right now. According to the American Heart Association, approximately half a million victims die from heart attacks every year. Two hundred and forty thousand are women. Strokes claim the lives of eighty eight thousand women and forty three thousand die from breast cancer yearly. These figures are constantly changing. They've been on a gradual incline over the years, with heart disease at the top. Although it may take ten or more years to affect women compared to men, it is clear that heart disease will continue to be our number one killer. Women usually develop heart disease during the time they've been more concerned about breast cancer and menopause. This is often the distraction that prevents women from seeking medical attention early enough to save their lives. After menopause most women's risk for heart disease begins to climb right up there with men. This is primarily because our estrogen level drops after menopause. Estrogen protects us from heart disease by its ability to increase our high-density lipoprotein levels (HDL). Women need more focus on heart disease prevention after menopause. Heart disease is frequently more fatal in women than it is in men. In this new millenium women's lives have become just as stressed compared to men. Stress is now an occupational hazard for women. We're holding high stressed positions in addition to taking care of older parents This increased level of stress is contributing to women's heart disease. In general men tend to survive their heart attacks, while women succumb.

High Cholesterol

A HIGH CHOLESTEROL DIET is the biggest danger to our blood vessels. Without patent (open) vessels the supply of oxygen and nutrients cannot be delivered as our cell demand them. On a cellular level our bodies will be deprived. This contributes to premature cell death and an acceleration of the aging process. During exercise we will receive insufficient oxygen supply. A poor oxygen exchange will contribute to: shortness of breath, excessively high heart rate, dizziness and difficulty developing physical endurance. Coupled with a sedentary lifestyle blood vessel diseases such as cholesterol plaque build up in our arteries are directly connected to saturated fats and animal products in our diet. We must cut the saturated fat, and the cholesterol connection to our diet in order to live free from the cardeo-vascular disease process.

Diet and Lifestyle

Diet and lifestyle are big players in our development of obesity, breast cancer, high blood pressure, heart disease, heart attacks and strokes. They are bigger players than our genetics. Modifications in our lifestyle can curtail, reverse or erase most of these preventable health problems.

Lack of Exercise

Lack of exercise coupled with poor diet is a large liability. Exercise is as necessary as food, air and water for a overall health. Exercise significantly improves our oxygen and carbon dioxide exchange rate. We need to exercise at eighty percent of our capacity in order to receive full benefits. However we should be able to carry on a conversation while exercising while being able to breath. Daily exercise is necessary if we're out of shape and or a candidate for heart disease. We're all candidates, but some of us are more vulnerable. We must use our knowledge and inner strength to ward off danger. A sedentary style of life is out of fashion in this new millenium. Action is our new style.

Obesity

Obesity is really a condition of excess adipose tissue (fat). It is a chronic condition of weight cycling (repeated gain and loss of weight). It's closely connected to genetics and biological components. Obese American women are at a higher health risk solely because they're obese (carrying at least 20 lbs. of excess fat). The 1988 report on nutrition and health estimated that one-fourth of adults Americans are overweight. Women with this condition can gain control over the cycling by being overly patient, dedicated and persistent in practicing a healthy lifestyle. This lifestyle should include regular low or non-fat foods, daily aerobics and stress management. Most obese women mistakenly focus only on counting calories, while neglecting their caloric output. The only way to control the weight fluctuation cycle is to carefully balance intake with output. Daily aerobics in the beginning is vital in improving pulmonary and cardiovascular (heart-lungs) capacity, while helping to burn calories. A slow and gradual increase in activities is key to increasing the metabolic rate and keeping a balance on our food intake and energy expenditure. Setting a goal to burn off one pound of fat at a time is realistic. 3,500 calories is equal to one pound. By simply walking moderately for 30 minutes a day we could burn off 1400 calories. In this way anyone can burn off a pound in less than three weeks. Losing excess fat very slowly is the most successful way for a chronically obese individual. Small loses of even 10% of initial weight will have significantly improve risk factors such as: hyperlipidemia (excess fat in the blood), blood sugar imbalance, high blood cholesterol, joint pain, and physical and emotional stress. Medical consultation should be sought, as part of our weight loss program. With every inch of fat a woman gains her chances for breast cancer also increases. A high fiber, low fat, high complex-CHO diet with regular exercise and group interaction therapy is said to be a very strong program in controlling obesity over time. Commercial weight loss programs have not been successful in controlling obesity. The regain cycle occurs about six months to one year. Some women may need medical treatment in conjunction to lifestyle changes. A physician with expertise in weight management is the right place to start seeking help. All the while never giving up your own knowledge and personal power to take charge of your health. In the long run only the very highly motivated individuals are able to maintain their weight.

Diabetes

Chronic diabetes is connected to obesity, and various cardiovascular problems. These conditions can be controlled with diet, exercise and available drugs if indicated. Diagnosed diabetic should make sure to keep their blood sugar under control. If medical treatments are necessary they should seek it.

Dietary And Emotional Stressors

Some diets are stressful on our bodies and are difficult to digest. Prolonged internal dietary stress leads to many gastro-intestinal diseases such as ulcers and acid reflux disease. Internal stress influences how we cope with external stress. It causes our bodies to become tense. We enter into the fight or flight syndrome when we're stressed. Good nutrition, regular exercise, and mental and spiritual relaxation are preventive and curative approaches to stress. These practices should be carefully incorporated into our contemporary stressful lifestyle in a pro-active attempt to prevent related diseases.

The Connection Between Pregnancy and: Diet, Fitness and Our Heart

Our hearts probably work the hardest when meeting the demands of pregnancy. During pregnancy, the mother's blood volume increases over fifty percent. It also assures the nourishment and survival of the baby. Most of us, if not all of us can survive several pregnancies with no fear of heart attacks by living a healthful lifestyle. A pregnant mother who regularly exercises, and eats as we've discussed will stay in good shape and good health. We can have big hearts and we can do great things without getting an enlarged weak heart. We're called the weaker sex, but perhaps we're really just wiser. Our best show of wisdom is to take charge of our health. We have the silent inner source of strength and courage to face facts. We know that without a fit inner and outer body we cannot carry out our function as women. With our mental fitness, and our spiritual will we're able to look truth in the eye and win. In the words of Shakespeare, " This above all, to thy own self be true." If you're a queen of denial it's time to snap out of it. Snap into courage, commitment and change for our future (our kids).

The Connection Between Fat and Breast Cancer

No more mastectomy; let's pro-actively practice **fat-ectomy, self breast-exams and have yearly clinical breast exams and mammograms**. Let's save our own lives ladies. Excess fat intake coupled with obesity after age thirty can significantly increase our risk for breast cancer. In the old days our grandmothers with breast cancer perished due to a lack of knowledge. Today much is known about cancer detection and prevention. With dietary measures, physical fitness and early medical intervention, we can escape breast cancer. Western women have the highest incidence of breast cancer in the world. Many researchers believe that fact is closely related to our **low fiber, high fat diet**. We can reduce some of the risk with a **low-fat, high fiber diet**. This type of diet reduces our estrogen level. A reduced estrogen level is a reduced risk for breast cancer. There are no guarantees in life. I must also point out to you that a low estrogen level could contribute to the development of heart disease. Some women with a history of heart disease benefit from estrogen replacement therapy. This is an area that you would need to discuss very carefully with your doctor in terms of the benefits or risks to you. What ever we need to do to stay healthy and to prevent diseases, lets begin with boldness today. Ladies I'm in this struggle with you for the long haul. Keep in mind that "The journey of a thousand miles begins with one step" (Chinese proverb). Lets mentally, physically, spiritually and consciously step into health. Let's leave all our troubles behind.

Chapter 8

Fitness For Fun, Freedom, And Great Health

It's time for us to work our own fitness alchemy and turn our bodies into genuine gold. Be sure to check with your doctor first.

Are You Ready for an Oxygen Transfusion?

What does aerobics do to Fat? "Burn, Burn, Burn. Aerobics is forcing our cells to utilize and burn oxygen at a greater rate; this action is good for overall health and fitness. It's the mother of metabolism boosting. Can we train our hearts to love us and not attack us? Yes. Aerobics can tame our hearts and make them user friendly, when it's connected to a healthy diet. Together they can turn any untamed heart into an angel of love. Do you want to keep your metabolism boiling hot, guzzling calories, and burning fat? Aerobics can do that for us. But what about bodybuilding? Can body building help women develop muscles that say fit, fun, and feminine? Certainly. Would you like to prolong your fountain of health with the exercise techniques of a champ? In this chapter I will share some of my pearls with you about how I went from motherhood and being overweight to becoming fit, fun, and fabulous. Aerobics and weight training can be used to tone, strengthen, and build muscles. They can also keep us youthful, vibrant, and healthy. The question is, are you ready to claim back your health. Getting you started is the principal focus of this chapter. Here is the list on exercising:

- Exercising
- Good News About Exercising
- Exercising Without Dieting
- A Story Is Worth A Thousand Words
- Check With Your Doctor
- Adding Exercise To Your Life
- Plan Ahead
- Where Do We Begin
- What Activity Is Best For Us

- Stretching The Secret To Staying Young Is To Stretch And Remain Flexible
- Thirteen Advantages Of Exercise
- Female Body Types And Responses To Exercise
- Genetic Body Types And How They Affects Us
- Muscles Can Be Feminine, Savvy And Sensational
- Pre-Exercise Pep-Talk
- Aerobics
- Why Will We Burn Fat And Not Muscles

Excercising

Whatever your reaction is to exercise, I believe you will come to appreciate and respect its benefits. Let's face the facts! The jury has deliberated and the verdict is unchallenged. It is unanimously agreed upon that exercise and diet are the two most important methods that we all need to get fit and healthy. They must be combined to get us through the long haul. Anyone can lose weight with diet or exercise, but it's impossible to keep it off without the two together. This is the life-sustaining couple from heaven, even though some of us feel like hell when we must eat right and exercise regularly. Remember there is a purpose to this pain. No pain no gain is only one way to see this, but when we find the why, we can deal with the how. No matter how difficult this process is, there are reasons why it's worth doing. One of my reasons is to live long enough to enjoy my grand- kids and to help mold their lives. If we're healthy and strong we're smart enough to appreciate what we have. We certainly wouldn't want to lose this precious gift from lack of regular exercise and a healthful diet. These benefits are the best insurance policy we can invest in. We will all get great returns. It's not like the stock market; there are no risks involved, and whatever we invest will increase. Lack of exercise coupled with a poor diet is a monumental risk to take with our one and only life. This risk could ruin our health permanently. It's like a slow ticking time bomb, all the while we're thinking that we're okay. A heart attack could be just around the bend, yet we have no apparent symptoms. Action is what makes the heart grow stronger. Today is the perfect time to build a healthful foundation in fitness. The only sure defense is offence, we must pro-act instead of re-act to stressful diseases. We all need to take action towards health and fitness and not wait to be treated because we have become ill, unfit or out of shape. We must assume an attitude of gratitude just to be able to take charge of our lives and our purpose. Every day I am more and more grateful just for having the gift of life. I go as far as picturing myself as an old woman to see the advantages of my present work in action. Are you ready to invest in your retirement? With my appreciation and respect for life I gladly make my daily deposits in my health and fitness account.

Good News About Exercising

With regular exercise, the death rate drops dramatically due to cardiac (heart) strengthening and increased endurance. We all know that heart disease is the number-one killer among Americans. On the other side of the coin is that our hearts can be user friendly. The more we use them, the friendlier, healthier, and happier they get. It's truly our best friend. We can't live without it, and we can't leave home without it. Our hearts are so kind they will respond warmly to any form of exercise we love. Any movement is better than a sedentary life style. Mr. Exercise and Mrs. Nutrition are the couple to save us from the serial killers Mr. Cholesterol, and Mrs. Fat.

Exercising Without Dieting

Exercise alone cannot undo the damage done by a high- cholesterol, and high-fat diet. In fact it can't break the bonds of fat and the plaque of cholesterol. If there were a choice between diet and exercise, we would probably lose more weight with diet alone. However, combining exercise with diet, simultaneously, is the best connection we can make. It's necessary to keep our BMR high, which is how we lose and maintain, our weight. We increase the speed and lasting benefits of ideal health and fitness, as well as weight loss and weight stabilization, when we completely connect in our minds that we must keep our diet and exercise as a team.

Marcia Sheridan, R.N.

A Story is Worth a Thousand Words

Let me share with you the story of a lady I'll call Susie. She neglected her physical appearance after her baby was born. She thought she would always have a husband to love and support her. For a while, her destiny was in incubation, and, then, what had not happened in years, happened in a day. She found herself divorced with a toddler to raise by herself. I'll never forget how she let herself go. Her outgoing personality, and magical magnetism had lost its charge. Her self-esteem shrank, while her waistline expanded. Her arms wagged like tails, and her thighs and buttocks were very shaky. Susie hated to exercise, but she loved to eat. Finally, out of desperation, she had some lipo-suction on her buttocks, inner and outer thighs, topped off with a pair of breast implants. Six weeks later, after the swelling went down, I took a look at her body. My eyes popped wide open, and my mouth dropped. I just couldn't believe what I saw. Before she took her clothes off, she looked nice and thin. But with her support stockings and tight jeans off, she looked like one of my geriatric patients. She didn't have flab hanging. She had skin hanging. I had never seen a post lipo-suction patient before. I was in shock.

She said to me, "I tried the easy way out, and now I have an old lady's butt. I guess I should have tried working out first. Well, the damage is done, I'll have to do the best I can now!" I was moved by her willingness to accept the consequences of her actions. I patted her on the back and said, "If you can come over on your free time, I'll show you how to build and tone up your muscles to help condition you." She started right there, asking me to do a workout with her in her kitchen. This was a woman who really hated to exercise and had never tried it before. It's never too late to take action. Plastic surgery does not rid us of our responsibility to eat and exercise properly. I was so proud of Susie when she finally accepted this fact. A fit and toned physique is the best surgery of all. Remember that all that glitters is not gold. Even if we're able to deceive people when we are wearing clothes, we may want to get undressed, at some point, in front of somebody. Furthermore, we all know what we really look like. It's not so easy to deceive ourselves totally, even if we're in denial. At some level, we know the real deal. Like my friend Susie, you, too, can start right now to reverse the gravitational pull on your body by doing your homework. Working out with weights will develop muscles under loose or sagging skin. If you already have a tight body, you are fortunate. You can maintain it with body toning and proper nutrition. We all succumb to the gradual wear and tear internally and externally. As we age, our muscles will atrophy due to insufficient usage and the normal aging process. It is a fact that most people tend to lessen their activities as they age. After the 20s, as we age, small amounts of muscle mass are lost, along with strength. This is the norm; however, I know from experience that building muscles can slow this process. My weight is about 95 percent lean muscle compared to my body fat, which was 5 percent. As a teenager, my body fat was approximately 22 percent even though I weighed only 105 pounds. I attribute the dramatic change in muscle-fat ratio to aerobics, weight lifting, and my new eating habits. My muscles have been the anti-gravity forces that have kept me looking youthful and vibrant. I expect my middle age (45-60) to be the best years of my life physically. I highly recommend bodybuilding with weights and aerobic exercise. Bodybuilding is not just weight lifting. It's any exercise that helps to build or tone your muscles. Anyone who exercises for health and fitness is a body-builder. When they hear the words "female body-builder," most people have a picture of women with enormous muscles that look like Arnold Schwarzenegger. That's not what I'm advocating. That's not what I was. I was a natural, drug-free, female body-builder. I've entered drug-free contests and was the first lightweight (106 lbs.), overall winner of the first Ms. Natural California. I also won the Ms. Natural All-American Female title. Keep in mind that I did all this after I had gained over sixty pounds during my pregnancy and four years after my son was born. My motivation to work out was just to get back in shape. Going from motherhood to Ms. America (for short) was an unexpected plus. Along the road of life, as women, we may lose our spouses and even our children, but there will always be you in your life. We need to try to accommodate ourselves, always, even if we have to make sacrifices or put ourselves first sometimes. The only person we can really expect to spend the rest of our lives with is ourselves. Make the extra time you need to do your workout. You deserve a workout today, so go for it. Become fit, fun and free.

Check With Your Doctor

Before you begin an exercise program, please see your doctor. Get a medical and physical evaluation that clears you for an exercise regimen. Be sure to inform your doctor of the intensity and type of workout you plan to follow, so that you can be advised professionally and appropriately based on your physical capabilities and health.

Adding Exercise to Your Life

It is important to get started with the right frame of mind. Regular exercises don't really build character or just build body. They reveal both, both of which were always there. Be realistic about your abilities and don't overdo your workouts. In the beginning, some of us are so headstrong we almost try to kill ourselves instead of help ourselves. We get stuck with temporary enthusiasm (temporary insanity) that burns out even before we lose one pound or tone one muscle group.

Plan Ahead

Failing to plan is planning to fail. When we fail to set aside time and means to exercise daily, it becomes easier by the minute to miss our work out. We're meaning to, but never getting to it. We struggle with the before feelings of "I hate it" or "I'll get to it next." Planning ahead puts us in charge. If we follow what we took time to plan, the after feeling is "I love it, I did it, I am more fit, I had fun, and I feel free".

Where Do We Begin?

We begin at the beginning. We begin with what we have. Maybe all we have is fifteen minutes worth of energy or only twenty minutes to spare. We can work with that. If we're able to walk fifteen minutes, we can add five more minutes to make it twenty minutes. Being consistent is the key, walking fifteen to twenty minutes every day or every other day is better for building up and maintaining our body than to run two miles every two weeks. It is the things we do regularly (whether good or bad for us) that make the difference in our lives, like making us fit or fat. By adding small increments to our exercise program, we will continually improve our fitness level. Adding variety by alternating the activities we love makes exercising more fun and challenging.

Which Activity Is Best for Us?

Any of the following sports can provide us with aerobic fitness: aerobic classes, swimming, walking, golfing, dancing, bike riding, tennis, baseball, roller skating, hockey, trampoline, jogging, or any physical activity that we enjoy, even team sports. An aerobic exercise is any exercise that stimulates the use of oxygen and one's heart and lungs to work hard enough to burn oxygen and calories. We must work up to 80% of our capacity in order to raise our metabolism and keep it high enough to burn fat. We must be able to keep up with our intensity level for at least twenty to thirty minutes in order to get the full benefit. Our intensity level is more essential in raising our BMR than our duration is. However, even ten minutes of exercise can be beneficial to our heart muscle. When choosing an exercise, remember that it is easier to maintain it if we have a passion for it. We need not feel that we have to be a professional athlete to participate in, and benefit from, different sports. To maximize the benefit of sports, we must first focus on preventing injury to the body through proper warm up and stretching.

Marcia Sheridan, R.N.

Stretching
The Secret To Staying Young Is To Stretch And Remain Flexible

Have you noticed in general that kids are very flexible while old people are very contracted, rigid and inflexible? Flexibility is definitely an antidote to old age, no matter how old you are. As we get older we become more prone to falls and broken hips. I have seen more old ladies die from infections due to inflexibility, falls, and fractured hips than any other accidents. Before stretching, it's a good idea to take a hot shower or bath or take a brisk, three-minute stationary walk to warm up the muscles. We need to remember to always stretch our muscles after warming them up. It is essential that we stretch for at least five minutes at the beginning of any exercise program. Stretching allows our bodies to prepare for the workout. It also decreases the chances of injuries. It is the quickest and easiest way to promote and improve flexibility, coordination, and balance. Regular stretching enhances the elasticity and strength of muscle groups. Stretching helps us to reach a little farther than our grasp by lengthening and improving the flexibility of our tendons. Begin stretches gently and slowly. Increase the tension of the stretch gradually until you begin to feel a slight resistance. Then, ease the tension and relax while holding the stretch for ten seconds. Repeat the same stretch again for ten more seconds. Never bounce or jerk while stretching and never stretch to the point of pain because one can tear or strain tendons and muscles. Ladies, if you wear high heels, stretch your calves before and after exercises. This will maintain elasticity, build stamina, and help prevent cramping in the calves. The trick to a great stretch is to avoid bouncing. Instead, hold the stretch. Stretching is also great for before, during and after pregnancy fitness and recovery.

Stretch to Cool Down: It is also recommended that we stretch at the end of our workout when cooling down. After every exercise routine, one ought to spend the last few minutes cooling down the body by stretching again. The cooling down phase allows the heart to return to a resting phase slowly. Abruptly ending the workout is stressful to the heart and other muscles. The easiest way to cool

CONNECTION COMPLETE

down is to gradually slow our movements. Finish the cool down period on the floor by stretching, while you inhale and exhale slowly, deeply, and completely. Stretching also includes the mind. As we stretch our bodies we do the opposite with our minds, we relax and calm the mind. We concentrate on each stretch and try not to let our thoughts wander away. Stay within the boundaries of your body—thus creating a true mind and body experience. In doing this we allow our stress level to decrease. Our minds also get a chance to rest and rejuvenate. Yoga is good for stretching our bodies while relaxing our minds.

Thirteen Advantages of Exercise
1. Control weight (fat in particular).
2. Increase Basal Metabolic Rate, (BMR).
3. Increase energy level.
4. Increase the production of white blood cells.
5. Fight infections and other pathogens.
6. Increase endorphin level and lift mood and PMS.
6. Improve the metabolism of glucose.
7. Reduce the risk of brittle bones and osteoporosis.
8. Lower our cholesterol level.
9. Reduce risk of heart disease and cancer.
10. Boost our immune system.
11. Increase self-respect and self-esteem.
12. Give us muscles to escape the JFJ.
13. FINALLY EXERCISE IS THE BEST SELF-PRESCRIBED STRESS REDUCTION PROGRAM WE COULD EMBRACE.

Marcia Sheridan, R.N.

Female Body Types and Responses to Exercise
Here are four distinct basic body structures

Type A Or Pear Shaped Structure

The **Type A** structure: is the typical narrow-shouldered, wide-hipped female. This structure is the most common of the four. They usually complain of gaining most of their weight below the waist. Weight training will help in toning their lower body, while building up their upper body. The method of high repetitions with light (5lbs-15lb) weights, is ideal for the lower body. It builds strength and stamina. It also helps to tone the upper body.

Type X or The Hour Glass Shape

The **Type X** structures: is the ideal structure for women. These women are usually well balanced, with strong shoulders, a small waist and strong hips and thighs. Most female athletes fall into this category. The X structure can benefit from all sports, including weight training. Women can trim or build up their upper or lower body depending on their preference, while keeping the waistline firm and trim. These divas proportions will always fall into place.

Type H Or The Straight Structure

The **Type H** structure: these women are athletically strong, maybe even stronger than the Type X structure. However they have a challenge with their waistline. This is their trouble area. They carry most of their excess fat around their waist. Aerobic exercises are helpful in trimming their waistline. Waist twisting and stretching is necessary to lengthen and trim the waistline. Some light workouts in weight lifting can help to tone the overall body. A good low fat diet can be very instrumental in trimming unwanted fat, to get that X appearance. This technique brings out the feminine beauty of the type H physique.

Type T

The **Type T** structure. These women tend to have strong shoulders, with an accumulation of fat around the waistline. From the hips down they are leaner and smaller in proportion to their upper body. This structure is very strong, especially in the upper body. Weight training could help these women to build up their lower body, and trim and tone their upper body. This approach combined with aerobics to trim the waistline, could help to balance the type T body structure nicely. Many people have a combination of two of the above four structures. With proper diet, exercise, work-out techniques, and wardrobe all four types can be bombshell beauties.

Genetic Body Types And How They Affect Us

1. ***Ectomorphs***: these individuals are slender. They have difficulty gaining weight no matter what or how much they eat. The body structure is more linear, delicate and less muscular. Weight training could be their lifesaver, in terms of building, and filling out their physique.
2. ***Mesomorphs***: these individuals will gain weight gradually, depending on their eating habits. The largest percentage of people falls into this group. They're well proportioned individuals compared to the other two groups. They gain weight or maintain their weight based on their diet and activity level.
3. ***Endomorphs***: these individuals gain weight easily. The mere sight or smell of food will stimulate their appetites. Endomorphs salivate at the sight of food. They love to eat. Endomorphs are usually burdened with excess weight.

No matter which of these categories we fall into, there is an exercise technique, and diet that can improve our health and physical ability. Next, I will discuss aerobics and weight training. Based on what you've just read determine which category (body type) you fit into, and follow the suggested exercises for you.

Muscles can Be Feminine, Savvy, Sexy And Sensational

Women often express some fear of lifting weights. They view weight lifting as a man's exercise. With this view, some women believe that, if they get into weight lifting, they will build muscles, and lose their feminine allure. This is not true. Women can build nicely toned feminine looking muscles using the toning technique of higher repetitions and lighter weights. Female hormones regulate how much muscularity a woman can develop. The average female who works out with the heaviest weights possible will still be unable to build muscles as large as the average male. This fact is directly related to the hormonal differences between the sexes. Genetics is another determining factor in how large your muscles can get. Some women genetically will be more muscular without ever having to lift weights. In this case, bodybuilding would only emphasize what was already there. Bodybuilding gives us the option of toning down our muscle size or building them up, depending on what we desire. Aside from the genetic differences between the sexes, my feeling is that tenderness and sensitivity are not only for women; nor are money and muscularity only for men. A muscular woman can be attractive, as can a sensitive man. We're living in a new age that is less gender specific and more spiritually conscious. I believe that in this new millenium we're ready to transcend such limiting beliefs. It's time to celebrate our spiritual unity and our mental ability while we build our physical body. Some of the most attractive females are athletic and muscular. As a matter of fact I find the Olympic female athletes to be very healthy looking, mentally strong and physically attractive. Female athletes never compromise their femininity although they have muscles. Muscles can lift our breasts as well as our buttocks, and tuck our tummy better than a plastic surgeon's knife. This will work for men and women alike. I think there is a nice balance in the fitness arena between men and women's appearance. We're into the new millenium; women are more sophisticated and are looking for more ways to exercise and eat to improve their health and appearance. Women are looking for more effective and quicker ways to tone their bodies and keep their attractiveness way into their later years. There is less talk about growing old gracefully. Boomers today want to remain beautiful. We need not be an Olympic athlete or a competitive female body builder to enjoy the strength, fitness level, and allure that a little muscularity can bring to our body.

Pre-Exercise Pep Talk
Put away the junk foods for a little sex appeal.

The fat burning mechanism of exercising can keep the appetite at bay for a while. We may notice that when we sit around doing nothing, we feel like eating more. When the urge to cheat creeps up (once a month at a certain time), I accept my humanity. I become proactive by taking charge and changing my behavior. I just grab a bottle of water and jump on my bike and I'm back on track. It's not what happens to us, it's how we respond that matters in the end.

Aerobics

Aerobic exercises cause the body to absorb large quantities of oxygen. This meet the respiratory requirements placed upon us by our increased use of muscles and increased cardiac output (heart rate). When our body is in a state of aerobics, it's in a state of burning oxygen and CHO (carbohydrates) for energy. In this state, the metabolism is elevated and maintained at a steady rapid rate. Although cardiovascular and respiratory rates are functioning at an accelerated pace, we should still be able to breathe adequately. If we become short of breath, we need to decrease our intensity level. Aerobic exercise is a fast way to increase stamina so we can endure the stress on our muscles longer. It helps to tone and strengthen muscles, improve respiratory functions, and strengthen and maintain our cardiovascular (heart) fitness.

Twenty minutes to one hour of continuous motion at our individual pace will improve:
1. cardiovascular fitness,
2. endurance
3. add tone to skeletal muscles
4. maintain body weight.

If we work out longer we will begin to burn fat. For best results these exercises should be combined with proper diet. It takes about an hour for the body to deplete its sugar source and its glycogen storage in the liver. After both sources of energy are depleted, fat begins to be burned to provide energy. For some people, it could be less than an hour. We're not expected to work out for an hour straight every time we work out. However, every little bit counts. Even if we don't burn fat, we're improving our cardiac fitness and toning. We still move up the fitness ladder by doing something.

Why Will We Burn Fat and Not Muscles?

Whenever our muscles are being stressed regularly, the body tends to rebuild and repair them as fast as possible. We lose our muscles only when we don't use them. In using our muscles we lose fat. We lose fat when we burn it as our energy source. In the constant use of our muscles, our body will finally realize that it has to set its thermostat to burn fat for energy. It also re-builds and repairs muscles faster under such stress. With this higher metabolism we usually tone and build muscle depending on the technique we use. Muscle toning and fat burning go hand in hand. At this stage, our body burns more calories even at rest. The rapid twitching of our muscles accelerates energy expenditure. This is the exact opposite of what happens to us when we go on starvation diets.

In a Nut Shell

The more we stress our muscles, the stronger they become, the stronger they become the longer our endurance becomes and we'll burn extra calories. Increased calorie expenditure, increases fat burning. The flip side of this coin is, the fewer calories we burn the more our metabolism will decrease. A low metabolism stimulates fat storage. The fatter we become the greater our risk for health problems, such as heart disease, heart attacks, obesity, breast cancer, stress, and premature death.

With proper diet, weight training and aerobics, our weight loss will not mean a loss of muscle fiber but a loss of fat. This is why weight resistance is so instrumental in fat loss. Weight training is the best way to strengthen muscles by creating resistance on them.

CONNECTION COMPLETE

Complementary to aerobic exercises, when combined with weight lifting, we can develop strength, muscle tone and muscle mass, improve our cardiovascular system, decrease our stress level, increase our self esteem and improve our total health and fitness body, mind, and soul. Because of the difference we can make in our physique and the speed at which it can be done, I highly recommend weight training. It is instrumental in preventing weak bones and osteoporosis. It has changed my life in a positive way that I never dreamed possible. I have not included before and after pictures because I don't believe they really show the dynamics of movement in between the start and finish. There is a lot of room for errors and poor techniques. Therefore I will do a video some time after this book to demonstrate my techniques. Stick with me ladies we're all in this together for the long haul.

Chapter 9

The Super Mom Work-Out

Getting in Top Shape Before and After the Baby.

These exercises are safe to do on your own providing you follow the instructions. "Marcia went from motherhood to Miss Fitness America. How did I do it?" I'll share that with you next. So let's see what we have in store for mom in this chapter:

- Before you move a muscle
- Post Delivery Isometrics, Toning and Strengthening
- Kegel Exercises For Your Pelvic Region
- Abdominal Exercises
- Abdominal Toning
- Pelvic Rock And Roll
- Pelvic Rocking On Your Hands And Knees
- Leg Exercises
- Derriere toning
- Back Rounding And Stretching
- Abdominal Oblique Stretching
- Waist Twisting
- Arms and chest Toning
- Stationary Bicycling
- Resistive Rebounding Exercises On The Trampoline
- The Mother Baby Connection Exercises

This chapter can be for ladies who desire to begin with a gentle program of fitness. It is, however, here specifically for ladies who are new moms, or maybe even those pregnant now. Ladies, this chapter can be instrumental in helping your body to bounce back. It's an easy and safe way to get back on the fitness track.

Before You Move a Muscle

Get your doctor's approval before you begin exercising. In all likelihood it's OK, but it's always wise to confirm your intentions with your doctor. When in doubt, check it out.

The next step is to keep the following precautions in mind as you begin your journey back to normal. Don't strain your body. Don't do any exercise to the point of pain. Stop exercising if you feel warm, dizzy, faint, nauseated, have a temperature, or have heavy bleeding. Avoid double-leg raises when in the supine position (flat on your back) and full sit-ups with legs straight (locked) in front of you. These exercises can strain the uterus and can cause heavy bleeding, especially in mothers who have had C-sections. These exercises can also hurt the lower back. Two or three short periods of exercise a day are safer than prolonged sessions that can cause strain and/or harm during the early post-delivery period. Now that we have discussed the little pit-falls of the possible early post-delivery complications, I think you're ready to actually start doing some simple exercises to regain strength and endurance and to improve your fitness level. You must be eager to fit into your old wardrobe. It's time to start picturing the way you desire to look, and feel, perhaps empowered, leaner, stronger, healthier, happier and more beautiful. I have been there, so let's do it together now.

Post-Delivery Isometrics, Toning, and Strengthening

The following exercises can be done immediately after delivery, even while you're in the hospital bed. Just ask your attending physician before you proceed. It's time to make a plan of action. Do it your way, and turn your future around by stepping in a new body, mind, and soul. Yes, at this point your body may be bruised, but it's not broken. So let's get started with the kegel exercise.

Kegel Exercise For Your Pelvic Region

This is the most important postpartum exercise a woman can do to repair some of the damage of childbirth. Kegels will strengthen and restore the most abused area of a woman's body during her delivery. The pelvic-floor musculature (the vaginal wall) is often left very bruised. Daily pelvic-floor exercises will help to restore the elasticity, tone, and integrity for future pregnancies. They help to prevent prolapse of the uterus (falling of the uterus down into the vaginal walls). Although I learned about Kegel exercises in nursing school, I couldn't really teach it to my patients from experience then, but now I can. I had lots of practice in my own classes but I really got the hang of it after I had my son. It makes such a drastic change in the body that you will want to master these exercises. As a matter of fact, after delivering a baby, you gain control of your vaginal muscles (that's what labor is all about). After giving birth, doing Kegel is a breeze and they're both worth doing. Arnold Kegel, a gynecologist, called attention to the pelvic floor exercises referred to as Kegel.

The action involved in Kegel is a tightening of the vaginal and abdominal muscles. Stopping and starting your flow of urine is a good way to familiarize yourself with these exercises. In the beginning, you may feel unsuccessful with these pelvic exercises. Don't be discouraged. These muscles have already been stretched, strained, weakened, and bruised to a very high degree depending on the difficulty of your delivery. If you persevere with the exercise, you'll gradually gain control and will show positive results. As you gain strength and control, try to hold the contractions a little longer. Use your abdominal muscles (abs) to exhale. Then let them relax and extend as you inhale. Then slowly exhale as you pull up and tighten your abs as well as your vaginal muscles. Hold it for a count of five to ten. The Kegel exercise is great for strengthening the pelvic walls and increasing the circulation to the perineum (vaginal area) which promotes healing in the episiotomy (small incision along the vaginal wall). It also speeds up the resumption of your intimate relations. The Kegel exercises can be done anytime, anywhere, and as often as you like. I still do them in my car at red lights. It gives me something positive to do, and it reduces stress on my lower back.

Abdominal Exercises

In the beginning of the post-partum period, the abdominal muscles are stretched, flabby, and loose. You may have some difficulty distinguishing between flab and muscle. The abdominal area seems like one or two big rolls of blubber. When you try to flex your muscles, it may barely move. It takes time to tighten up and contract into its proper place. The slower you lose weight, the more you lower your chances for stretch marks. Stretch marks become larger and more noticeable with rapid weight loss. Exercise helps to tone and tighten our skin, and pull it back into position. The safest approach after delivery for abdominal tightening can be done with an empty stomach in the supine position (flat back) as follows:

Abdominal Toning (Abs).

1. Inhale slowly and deeply letting your abdomen rise as you inhale laying flat on your back with knees bent.
2. Exhale slowly, contracting your abdominal muscles as tightly as you can while putting all of your weight on the small of your back.
3. Tuck your chin into your chest as you lift the shoulders and squeeze.
4. Hold this contraction for at least five seconds.

Repeat this technique for at least ten to twenty five times. Do this as often as you like. As you get stronger, and you're out of the danger of heavy bleeding (after you've stopped spotting), you can work the abs more vigorously. The diastasis recti (separation of abdominal muscles) can be corrected with these crunches (abdominal contractors). Strengthening your abs will take some pressure off your lower back, as well as give an elegant posture.

Pelvic Rock and Roll

Pelvic rocking is used to strengthen and to relieve lower backaches and improve posture:
1. Lie flat on your back with knees bent and legs shoulder-width apart.
2. Roll buttocks slightly forward as you tighten and squeeze the cheeks together, keeping your lower back on the floor or

bed. As you do this, exhale while tightening your abdominal muscles and pelvic floor muscles. Keep the small of your back flat on the floor.

3. Return to the starting position and repeat for at least five to ten minutes. Do this routine as often as you like.

As you get stronger you can do the same movements while on your hands and knees. It is an excellent way to kill two birds with one stone. You can combine the pelvic rocking, and abdominal tightening. Each movement can flow into the other, synchronized with your breathing.

Pelvic Rocking On Your Hands and Knees

This position will require more strength to tighten the abdominal muscles. Keep your back in straight alignment. While doing this, start rocking but do not allow your back to snap. All movements should flow smoothly like a symphony from one body part to the other, to avoid sudden, jerky motions and strains.

1. Position yourself on all fours. Position your palms under your shoulders and keep your knees under your hips.
2. Lower your chin to your chest. Tighten buttocks, squeeze abdominal, pelvic muscles as you exhale, pulling your lower back up towards the ceiling into a cat stretch.
3. Lift your head. Roll pelvis back and relax all muscles as you resume straight back position. Repeat for at least five minutes. Do this as often as you like.

Leg Exercises

Lay flat on your back, while bending one leg to support your back and abdomen, extend one leg at a time.

1. Flex your calf muscles.
2. Wiggle your toes and feet.
3. Flex your foot and point toes.
4. Then bend your foot back towards your face as far as possible until you can really feel the stretch.
5. Flex your foot from left to right and circle.

Alternate the same program with both feet three or four times. Do these two to three times per day for toning, strengthening, and as preparation for more vigorous exercises. Leg exercises while in bed also help to improve circulation and prevent the formation of blood clots.

Derriere Toning

This exercise strengthens the buttocks, abdomen, quadriceps (thighs), and lower back. It increases spinal flexibility. It should be done slowly, and smoothly.

1. Lie on your back with your feet about ten inches apart and knees bent.
2. Slowly squeeze and raise buttocks and the lower back. As you do this, contract abdomen and pelvic floor while you ex hale and hold for five seconds. At this point in the routine, your upper body should be flat and relaxed.
3. Inhale slowly as you return to the floor one vertebra at a time
and then relax. Continue doing this for five to ten minutes.
This movement will tone the buns and thighs.

These are exercises you can do when you are stronger and have been taken off bed rest by your doctor. By now you should also be able to prepare proper meals. This is the awakening phase of motherhood; when your future and your baby's life are on the road to being fit, fun, and free.

By this time you should be home, on your feet, and making the touchdowns. Let me inject a little nutrition here to help boost and expedite your fitness goals. First of all, take cues from the baby. If it eats only when it's hungry, so should you. Your newborn instinctively stops feeding when it's full and so should you. This is a good time to reconnect to your own instinct. The baby is getting a wholesome, healthful diet, so should you. Starting a new healthy lifestyle along with the new magic in your life is a great new start for both of you. Consume high-quality complex CHO, low-fat foods, lots of fruits and vegetables, and a whole lot of love from your baby. At the end of this book, you'll know how to put it all together. Back to stretching and warming up for the big times.

Back Rounding and Stretching

1. Start in an upright sitting position on the floor with knees bent and up against the chest with feet flat.
2. Slowly hug your knees and push your back away. Let your head drop forward as you extend your arms, almost locking your elbows. Tighten your stomach muscles and pelvic walls as you exhale. Round out the back completely and hold for five seconds.
3. Slowly pull chest back towards the knees. Lift the head and relax while you breathe freely. This is a great stretch for your back and arms.

Abdominal (Oblique) Stretching

1. Start in the standing position with feet apart and the arms and hands extended over your head in a clasped position. Tighten abdominal floor for support.
2. Curve your torso to the left without arching the back. Stretch the right hip up to the shoulders and move in a slight pull by the left arm and hold for five seconds.
3. Return the torso to center position. Relax and breathe. Re peat this motion on your right side. This will help loosen any spare tire you may be burdened with.

Waist Twists

This exercise helps the waist stay trim and flexible while strengthening and relaxing the lower back:
1. Lie in a supine position with arms stretched out to the sides with palms facing down and knees bent.
2. Keep shoulders flat on floor. Twist bent knees from the waist to the right until they touch the floor (or as close to it as

possible).

3. Return to center. Swing knees to the left and repeat for five minutes. You should also tighten abs and pelvis as you exhale and hold briefly at each twist. Repeat as often as you like from side to side gently.

Arms And Chest Toning

Beginner pushups: Do one to four sets of eight repetitions. This exercise is for those who can't do the full pushups.

1. Start with knees on the floor, with hands shoulder-width apart.

2. Bend elbows, touching chest to the floor (or close to) and pushing up to starting position.

3. Continue to do daily until you reach desired results, or until you're able to do the full push-ups.

4. If you're not able to do push-ups on the floor you could stand up and do the same movement against the wall until you build up enough arm (triceps) strength to do it in a horizontal position. Stick with it, ladies, it will certainly payoff.

Stationary Bicycling

Before you start riding, make sure that your episiotomy (incision) is well healed, and there is no chance of bleeding, or ask your doctor. To do this at home you need to have a stationary bike. It's an excellent investment and a big convenience to have at home. I adjust the speeds for different tension levels, and I work up to 90% of my capacity sometimes. I read, watch TV, and sometimes play catch-ball with my son Eric, while riding. This makes it less monotonous, and I can easily ride for an hour. I strongly recommend a stationary bike as the perfect addition to a home gym. Here are some benefits for an investment in a stationary bike. You can begin to get an increase of oxygen into your blood and a good dose of aerobic exercise. Aerobics means getting more oxygen into your blood. More oxygen, with a proper diet means faster fitness and faster restoration of your body, mind, and spirit. Since you haven't had much aerobic type exercise for a while, it will take a little while for you to build up to twenty minutes or more of riding. Persevere. Aerobics provides adequate oxygen to your brain, tissues, and circulation. It also stimulates our lymphatic system to get rid of toxins. This keeps our immune system healthy. Increased oxygen in the blood is vital for our cardiac endurance, cell rejuvenation, and our fitness level. A few other fringe benefits for new mothers, and women who want to be beautiful and alluring, are a healthy glowing appearance and a fresh feeling of aliveness and energy. A little aerobics and oxygen increase is also helpful in burning off those stubborn old fat cells that we've all gained during pregnancy.

Resistive Rebounding Exercise On The Trampoline

You don't have to be a gymnast to reap the benefits of the trampoline. Just in case you can't ride a bike, here is another chance to reap the same aerobic benefits. I tell you, ladies, working out in oxygen is the quickest connection to vitality. You can replenish your vitality and energy level any time you get a break. Just begin to move and breathe for at least twenty minutes at a comfortable pace. Use of a trampoline can help you develop your strength, balance, coordination, and endurance. I have been using a mini-trampoline to do my aerobic exercises since my back injury. By using a trampoline instead of running, or jumping up and down in an aerobic class, you can avoid excess force, constant jarring and pressure on the joints, which can result in injuries of the low back, knees, and Achilles tendon. Rebounding is ideal for people with chronic injuries. It's also another way just to add variety to your work-out and work the entire body. I include two half-pound wrist weights to increase resistance to upper body, while I use the bike for my legs. I alternate the trampoline with my bicycle routine from day to day. You will need sneakers with good support. I have been rebounding on my trampoline now for six years, and I have noticed an improvement in my coordination and flexibility. I find rebounding to be the best all-around aerobic activity for me. It's easy on my back and knees which is very, very important to me now. If you have an injury or arthritis, this is a way to keep moving and breathing aerobically without killing your joints. It is the next best thing to swimming. Be watchful when using it with kids.

The Mother - Baby Connection Exercises

This is a bonding exercise for mother and baby to have fun together. While you strengthen your thighs, it helps the baby to strengthen its neck, and support its own head. Your baby should be strong enough to arch its back and support its head. I enjoyed watching Eric laugh and act excited during this exercise. This was one that we both enjoyed immensely. It also helped him in his own physical fitness, and normal growth and developmental stage. The aging process starts at birth, so should the fitness process. Exercising together helps to strengthen the bond between a mother and her child. It is also a healthful thing to teach and to do together, so let's get start.

1. Start by lying flat on your back with knees bent towards your face. Have the bottom of your feet facing straight away from you.

2. Carefully place the baby in the prone (face down) position laying on your shins. Use your feet to support its feet while you hold the upper arms or hands.

3. Stretch your baby's arms out to the side while you raise your shins with feet slightly higher than your knees. Hold the position for five seconds, and then slowly return to the starting position. You and your baby will have so much fun that the two of you will want to continue exercising forever. This experience is like the best roller coaster ride ever for the baby. It makes mom out to be a symbol of love and pure pleasure. Moms, it's healthful, it's fun, it's fit, and it's freedom for both of you.

By this time, ladies, you shouldn't have any difficulty visualizing yourselves looking your best. Once you perceive it, and believe it, you will achieve it. Taking a view of the new you will help you to stay on the course and maintain your health, fitness and dignity. We have come a long way with our babies, our treasures in life. As a new mother and as a woman, we must vow to keep our kids out of the junk food jungle and keep them fit, fun, and free! By example we can do this. They'll have all of their lives to internalize and hone these skills. What a wonderful advantage and gift to give and to receive. Our kids deserve a healthy life, and so do we. Let's start a new age of being fit, having fun, and enjoying freedom that a healthy lifestyle has to offer. My spirit is with you mom. Let's all complete the connection together.

Chapter 10

Holistic Health and Harmony

Understanding the Mind-Body Connection from a Spiritual Point of View

Welcome to the renaissance of women's spirituality, a divine state of enlightenment whose time has come. A time to disconnect from our individual myopic mentality, cultural hallucination and emotional poisoning; and to completely connect to the elements of our being. This includes our physical health and fitness, mental consciousness, personality, sexuality, spirituality, and personal responsibility. It's time for a global makeover of female health and wholeness. In this chapter we'll talk about the following:
- The Connection Between Sexuality and Overweight In Women
- What's The Connection Between Women and Their Sexuality?
- Connecting To Our Inner Source Of Creation Through Visualization and Affirmation
- Manifesting Our Feminine, Social, Sexual and Spiritual Self.
- The Social and Psychological Stigmas of a Woman's Body Image.
- Affirmations
- Affirmations For Health and Happiness For Body, Mind and Spirit

Contradicting Our Common Sense As Intuitive Women Being

Most of us want a balanced life of health, happiness and purpose; but when it comes to our behavior, we do every thing to sabotage such a belief. We **STRESS** ourselves out every day. We have very little fun, and our idea of a balanced diet is a big-burger in one hand and a large fries in the other. At the end of all of that we say we don't want to get fat, we want to live a stress-free life, and we want to enjoy the good life. When, in fact, our lifestyle is lousy in every way possible. Such contradictions in our psyche bring guilt, stress, fear, anxiety and disease within our physical body. Such diseases eventually transmit destructive parasitic thoughts to our minds and potent poisons to our spirits, which we consciously and unconsciously transmit to our world. We do this through the character weaknesses and personality pathology that we have developed. We need to make a paradigm shift from our old mind set. We must stop confounding our common sense, confusing real issues in our lives and become conscious of the impact of our thoughts and interaction with self and others. I believe we're ready to stop kidding ourselves and to stop the duplicitous war within. I'm referring specifically to the war that goes on between our emotions and our spirit. This war within is a life-long battle that we often lose. We lose the war and gain the weight; the same old story over and over. Why? We all think of changing our little world around us, but we're slow to change ourselves. Why? Let's be wise and start with our inner selves first. All of the images we have of ourselves, namely: physical, mental, spiritual, social and sexual, is the core of our entire being. As women, we're determined to live completely connected to inner and outer dimensions, in order to experience the miracles of life. We'll enjoy our lives wholeheartedly by focusing our intentions on unconditional love, compassion, and forgiveness of ourselves and others. In addition to diet and exercise, we will practice giving ourselves a jolt of faith and courage every day. To experience total health, we must nourish our entire being. Our spirit also needs food and exercise to stay alive and wholesome. We're more of spirit than we are mortal. We will nurture our spirits and souls through prayer, meditation, visualizations, affirmations, and faith in our source of creation. We have been evolving magnificently juxtaposed to our male companions. However, we're "woman." We're of a different mental and spiritual make up. Therefore let us connect and celebrate the feminine mystique of our womanhood. On the other hand we are aware of our masculine side. It's a part of our wholeness. We understand what Hubert Humphrey meant when he said, "Never give up and never give in," because, as women, this sentiment is vital in our journey to wholeness. We, too, can flex our muscles and fight to the finish when we keep our eyes on our desire. What are your desires? What images of yourself do you desire and dream of? What image of yourself do you think would make you whole and beautiful inside and out? Harmonizing all the images we have of ourselves can really produce a richer and fuller life. A fuller life is not just physical health and fitness. It's when all of our component parts, internal and external, work in agreement for the completion of our authentic purpose in life. It's consciously connecting all the wonderful blessings that make us complete beings. The subject of diet and exercise has been on the front burner of our minds throughout this book. Let us now paint the portrait of a complete **woman being**. We must start with our authentic self, which is our real self, our inner core. We cannot allow the demise of our spirit by ignoring the inner world of our self. The beginning of our freedom, enlightenment, and self-actualization begins with a spiritual connection to our conscious self. That is true enlightenment within and without. Poverty of vision and poor knowledge of self is the enemy that has deprived us from genuine health and happiness. It has kept us as slaves to the junk food jungle, super-saturated in stress, and disconnected from our desires. In our contemporary culture of high stress, we all need to exercise our vision, knowledge, and power without losing our soul. Let us, now, deepen our insight into some of the struggles women wrestle with in terms of their femininity, their personal power as women, their size, and their value as people.

The Connection Between Sexuality and Overweight in Women

What woman in her right mind wouldn't want to be alluring and satisfied in all aspects of her being? We recognize our sexuality as essential and worthy of fulfillment in order for us to be complete. However it's a topic that has not been addressed from a spiritual perspective. We need to become more enlightened to the connection between sexuality and overweight in women. Let's take a closer look at our views on female sexuality, our body image, our self-esteem and the use of our body size to control our environment, protect us from the opposite sex, or to attract them to us. We want a healthy body, and we want to keep it too. Therefore we must end the battle within our hearts and minds that is slowly eroding our completion as total women beings. The good news is that we have the ammunition to end this war as winners. Since we must all take pride in our bodies as women, we can do this very diligently without turning away from our life's purpose. We begin by sending our self-destructive urges into the abyss and summon our spirit back. Let's say we only have an average or even below average figure. The truth is, whatever we have we should respect and appreciate totally. It's only when we're able to do this on a spiritual level, are we able to attract, from our source of creation, the best that it has in store for us. For a long time I was insecure about my body. I covered it with fine clothes to compensate. This was a superficial camouflage, and a quick fix approach. However after my son was born, I had to do much more than just hide myself under my clothes. But not to complain or self-destruct, I discovered proper diet and exercise techniques that work better than fashion camouflage, suction catheters, plastic surgeon's knives, fad diets and drugs. But by practicing the disciplined actions persistently to become totally healthy I became connected to my inner self. Through the initial physical approach I became connected to my emotional energy, intuition, and spiritual source of strength. These forces working in harmony with my divine purpose and desires, have kept me completely connected for the past sixteen years. I went from a **so-so physique** to an **Oo-la-la** physique that was fit, healthy and a pleasure to live in. I feel an overall sense of peace and harmony within and without. You too have now made the discovery of proper diet and exercise as well as your inner source of strength. It is time for you to weave a new tapestry of life. We can all be beautiful and alluring no matter what our external size. We know that we're not just a body size, but a complete being on a refining process towards completing our individual purpose. We need not be ashamed of our bodies. We must nurture them as the physical vessel of our journey and purpose on the planet. God gave women the gift of beauty in a physical form. We are bodies of divine beauty, not just physical. But being sexy, healthy and wise is part of the package. When we step into a— **what a beautiful healthy looking woman attitude**, we automatically appreciate and feel good about ourselves as people. Our spirit, self-image, and self-esteem jumps to life. We feel a magnetic force of spiritual and emotional vibrancy. In addition to proper diet and exercise, our feminine grace reveals the beauty of our character, and personality as individuals and as **women being**. I believe that inside of every woman is a loving and nurturing soul, a gift to be manifested to humanity and a sight of inner and outer beauty to behold. Isn't it worth digging deeply to discover and completely connect to **the beautiful female** hidden away from us, from our mental and spiritual eyes? Come on, ladies. Let's get enthusiastic with our gifts as **women being**. Start the digging within. We're worthy of such a divine treasure hidden within ourselves.

What's The Connection Between Women And Their Sexuality

Why be sexy? Why not be sexy? Why is not the point. The point is that we are. Our sexuality is a part of our spiritual, physical, and emotional expression of ourselves. Our sexuality is not limited to the physical act. It transcends it. Sexuality is energy that is uplifting to our entire being. When we feel comfortable with our sexuality, we also feel energized and high-spirited. We can be the most creative and productive when we experience our sexual energy. Most women are the most energized and creative when they're in love, with self or others. The energy of love is to connect and experience universal energy. It makes us feel alive and attractive, which makes us sexy. When we feel sexy, we are high on our own, natural endorphin and juices. We are nice to people, and to ourselves, when our sexual energy is overflowing. Sexual energy is a natural flow of inner vibrations that make us feel better than, drugs, alcohol, or the junk food jungle. Sexual energy is god sent, it's creativity, inspiration, self-love, and individual expression. We need only to understand this and to act wisely when we're in this state. This is an energy to be shared with divine purpose in mind. It is not to be abused for the selfish gratification of our carnal desires. The opposite sex is always drawn to our energy. Yes, most men will give their souls to a woman with such energy; especially our husbands incidentally. We won't need a sexy wardrobe to get their attention. Our radiation of energy and spirituality is a stronger magnet. It reveals to the world that we're feeling great. It's a great stress reducer and the key to attracting goodwill. As far as charming the opposite sex with our god given alluring beauty, we can present it with style. The most glamorous gifts we can present to our husbands are a sharp mind, self-love, confidence, and a healthy body. Let's put the men in our lives aside for a while. What other reasons are there for us to be alluring and feminine? We can be alluring for our emotional health and wellbeing. If we're not turned on by what we see in the mirror, how can we be at peace with our femininity. When we feel our femininity we're usually healthy, but we cannot be sexy when we're unhealthy mentally, physically or spiritually. In fact, we usually feel sexier and more feminine when we are in great shape. We even sleep better. We awake feeling rested and full of energy. We feel like running the world. When we look into our mirrors and see a reflection of health and fitness, we feel empowered and loved by ourselves and by the universe. When we love ourselves, others are spellbound to respect and appreciate who we are. Hopefully, we can start each day feeling great and looking great, with an attitude of gratitude for the gift of life. Such good vibes attract the right people to us who are healthy, positive people just like ourselves.

Connecting To Our Inner Source of Creation Through Visualizations and Affirmations

Are you ready to journey into your universe and discover the star you've never noticed before? We can begin by calmly reacquainting and connecting our spirits to this source. Being totally calm helps to bring inner peace and conscious connections within our body, mind and spirit. One way to benefit from our affirmations is to be totally honest with ourselves as we visualize and acknowledge our deepest fears, stress, intentions and love and forgiveness for self and others.

Here is my V-A (Visualization and Affirmation) program.
—*I see myself as the beautiful being that I am.*
—*I forgive myself for all my shortcomings.*
—*I forgive everyone who has offended or hurt me.*
—*I will use my thoughts and feelings as a path to self-actualization.*

—I will do things that lift my spirit and make me feel whole.
—I will always work towards my own peace and tranquility and take responsibility for my own happiness. I am totally grateful for my life as it is now.
—I will express my spiritual and sexual energy with divine wisdom.
—I will strive to be in harmony with myself and with the earth.

Manifesting Our Feminine, Social, Sexual and Spiritual Self

Given the fact that we are sexual beings, and that it's part of our God given spirituality, we should feel free to express sexuality in an **appropriate** and **natural** manner. It's not a part of ourselves we need to fear, or to exploit. Sexuality can be expressed in many different ways. We can express our sexuality through mannerisms, art, music, conversation, work, hobbies, entertainment, or fashion. Sexuality is just another expression of adult intimacy, according to Eric Erickson's school of psychology. Sexuality and intimacy appears primarily in the adult stage that he calls "Intimacy Vs. Isolation." This is not to say that if you're not intimate, you're going to feel isolated. The point is, just as it's paramount that we diet and exercise to enjoy health, we need to likewise express all aspects of our being to be in harmony with our inner and outer self. Sometimes we enter the junk food jungle because intimacy has exited our lives. We replace it with food, not healthy food but junk food, and lots of it. Being physically stressed can kill our spirituality and our sexuality. Our unexpressed need for intimacy turns into a desire to eat because that's easier, and it's also pleasurable. Some people turn to alcohol, drugs, or cigarettes, which perpetuates the cycle of stress and poor health. We know that this type of stress can leave us stuck in the city of obesity, heart disease and cancer. We know better, now, don't we ladies? In this new millenium we're expanding personal power and collectively widening our gender roles beyond motherhood. As women, we have pulled away from the stereotypical sex roles, the old social ideals of how women should express their femininity and how to behave appropriately.

Marcia Sheridan, R.N.

We now collectively express ourselves to the world as whole beings, showing our intellectual brilliance equally as much as we express our feminine finesse. Today we flex our muscles, change our own flat tires, pump our own gas, ward off sexual harassment, and bring home the bacon. At the same time we realize the obvious physical, mental and spiritual differences between men and women. We know our limitations and our vulnerabilities as women, and we're quick to acknowledge them. We also recognize that there are masculine and feminine traits in everyone and we chose to express them differently. Over the years we have learned that a little muscle will tone our bodies and make us stronger; while a high-fat diet can cause cancer and heart attacks. What can we do? Escape the junk food jungle and take charge of our lives. We're now willing and able to make the necessary changes to take charge of our lives, because we're no longer willing to sacrifice any aspect of our woman being. We will complete our connection spiritually and allow our purpose to blossom.

The Social and Psychological Stigmas of a Woman's Body Image

In our culture, body image is at the forefront of a woman's identity. Strong feelings about our bodies are woven into practically every aspect of our behavior. Whether we're fat or thin, we develop a body image based on how we're perceived. Body image certainly isn't all there is to being a whole person. But because we're judged by society mainly by our appearance we become disconnected from our inner self and completely fixate on our body image. We cannot escape the judgement of the physical eye, our culture have not evolved enough spiritually as yet; it is up to us to help bridge this gap. Our contemporary culture is still very visual, judgmental and youth-oriented. Because our bodies are the first, most instant, and visible means of presentation, our physical appearance is the standard to be judged by. We can still keep our sight focused on our internal purpose, while we convey a strong message with a healthy body—wherein our bodies, by themselves, are **the message** of who lives inside. Just as clothes make fashion statements and reflect social and financial success so, too, can one's strong posture, pleasing appearance and spiritual glow reflect total success. These nonverbal messages tell the world something of who we are long before we open our mouths. Don't believe people do not judge us by the way we look. Although they may not admit it, they do. People react to their perceived image; therefore our body image as women does have profound effects on our self-esteem, whether we realize it or not. Self-esteem can affect our attitudes towards every aspect of our lives. Knowing the power that our body image has on our overall feeling of self, one's appearance is also a reason to diet and exercise. Sometimes it's through our bodies that we connect with ourselves and with others. The less spiritual people are the more difficult it is for them to connect with us other than through their physical perception of what they see. We live in a sensory world where most people can't see beyond their five senses. Therefore it's wise for us to understand that, but not judge and persecute ourselves by such limited views. Nor is it wise to develop our self-image or body-image based on such external superficial limitations. We can recreate our image of self from a more spiritual source of wisdom. By dwelling on positive thoughts we will attract this source of power and change into our lives. We'll be able to take positive actions towards our thoughts with effortless gains. One way is through daily prayer, visualization, affirmations, and an honest desire to connect to our source of creation. I have noticed more peace in my life since I have adjusted my attitude and responses to external forces. For example, our attitude towards stress is what makes stress stressful, humorous, or exciting. Be willing to view stress with a spiritual eye. Look for the positive—look for the lessons to be learned. Positive affirmations are great ways to change our attitude, prejudices and behavior. I've noticed that when I keep positive thoughts, envision peace, satisfaction, and happiness, I always enjoy a big smile. My level of stress decreases and I realize it's a wonderful world. Our spiritual source of power is the nutritious cure of our weaknesses because it makes us strong and positive and it satisfies our true hunger in life. Consistent **visualization** and **affirmation** (**VA**) are ways to manifest continuous positive energy and events into our lives. With **VA**, we can experience an abundance of joy in living. VA's are **pain-free, struggle-free, and fat free**. It's a way of healing our soul and calling our spirits into consciousness. **Visualizations** work best within a quiet mind. I think we can all agree that our bodies are pieces of clay that are workable and shapeable. We can mentally create our image and connect them to our spirit. Like Michelangelo, we can create our own synergistic connection within and without. To use **VA**, we should focus on our blessings not our wants. We begin with gratitude for all our gifts, physical, mental, and spiritual. There is a lot of truth to the motto "Love thyself first." First of all, picture your source of creation as a loving and kind source. Enjoy the feeling of receiving its love. It's awesome. Then picture someone who once loved you or still loves you. Enjoy what it feels like to be loved by that person, to be cherished and adored. If there is no one, picture your favorite pet and how much it appreciates you. Think about the joy you get from cuddling your pet. If you don't have a pet, get one; they're god's gift of love to us. Begin to picture yourself as you really are. Then start your VA's giving thanks to the universal source of love. Use your own name. This is powerful stuff! Believe me. Here are a few to keep your mental and spiritual battery charged.

Affirmations

* I love and accept (substitute your own name) just as she is.
* I will honor and respect (add your name) as she is.
* I am very pleased and proud of the character (your name) has grown into.
* I enjoy meditating, and spending time alone with (your name).
* (Your name) character is strong, confident, supportive, consistent, persevering, kind, sensitive, generous, intuitive, wise, and humble.
* I love the way (your name) takes excellent care of herself mentally, physically, and spiritually.
* I think (your name) is a healthy, happy, and a very well adjusted-woman.
* I, (your name), will always try to give back to the planet by practicing "Age- old" advice: I will " do all the good I can,

by all the means I can, in all the ways I can, in all the places I can, all the times that I can, for everyone I can."

* (your name) diets and exercises for the betterment of her health, body, mind and spirit.

*(your name) is loved by nature, the universe, and herself.

Affirmations for Health and Happiness for Body, Mind, and Spirit.

Because you have taken charge of your health, you can rightfully affirm yourself:

* I desire to manifest whatever is wholesome and wise for me.
* I believe all things are possible for me.
* I believe that with the guidance of my divine source of creation I will always make the right decisions for my well being.
* I believe when I put my best into the universe, it will returns in abundance.
* I believe I can always be transformed by the renewing of my mind.
* I recognize the potential for growth and enlightenment in my daily life.
* I lay no blame, but will take full responsibility for all my own actions.
* I will forever moving in harmony, and peace with the universe.
* I will give of my possessions and myself generously, expecting nothing in return.
* Obesity is no longer a monster I fear. It does not exist in my body.
* Stress no longer has a rope around my neck.
* I can soar over mountains higher than Mount Everest.
* I have escaped the JUNK FOOD JUNGLE.
* I now have Complete Power and Control over my life's purpose.
* I am now FIT, FUN, and FREE.

CHAPTER 11

How Did I Complete My Connection To Total Health And Harmony?

Finding the Will, I went from being overweight, after motherhood to becoming Miss natural Fitness America.

- How Did I Completely Connect to Total Health and Harmony
- Island Girl Comes To Brooklyn N.Y.
- The Pregnancy
- Recovering From Pregnancy And Delivery
- Breast Feeding And My Weight Loss
- Japan: A New Awakening
- The Connection Payoff
- The Greatest Challenge

In order to give you a clear understanding of my journey through the jungle and how it has completely connected me to my entire woman being allow me to give you a brief background of the culture I came from. In my old culture life was simple and free. I learned to enjoy the bounty of nature, and to instinctively enrich my spirit with the source of my creation. Listening to the sparrows and the Jamaican Doctor birds sing, was a spiritual delight. When Christmas came and there was no gift under the tree, I could go to the beach and wash away my sadness in the great ocean of renewal. The clear blue sky, the tropical flowers, and the awesome sunsets were the gifts I learned to unwrap in my mind. Such natural abundance was like the earth, wind, and fire of my soul. In this chapter I'll share with you the change in my life after leaving a simple culture in Jamaica for one that's vastly more complex. A culture built on super- saturated-stress. I had to quickly learn all the skills to survive, thrive, and stay alive in America. I believe it will motivate you to take an inner trip to the island of complete connection that lies within all of us. My short life in Jamaica is one I can never forget. It's still a part of my soul, a part that I wish to share with you throughout this chapter. I was very in tune with nature. Even my heartbeat was in tune with the drums of the Reggae beat. Jamaica was the ultimate healthy habitat for humanity. Most Jamaicans lived off the land and the ocean without too much shedding of animal blood, pollution, or disharmony of our ecosystem. They have divine reverence for the rights of our ecological system to evolve naturally. Jamaicans understand and completely respect the interdependent connection between man and nature. Jamaicans live a low-stress, low-fat active lifestyle naturally; long before we knew the value. Their lives are much larger than their livelihood. They have the abundance of spiritual wealth connected in their hearts culturally. Certainly they do not have the affluence of Americans in terms of money, and standard of living, but they're very rich in their contentment, and love of a healthy and fit life. Lack of material things is not a source of stress, because they have very little wealth to warehouse as well as very little worries to stress over. Jamaicans find their wealth within themselves. We respond to conflicts with an attitude of "no problem man," "Respect."

How Did I Completely Connect to Total Health and Harmony?

Let me now tell you how I transitioned from fit, fun, and free, to fat, flabby, and flabbergasted, and then back to total health and harmony. Picking fruits, climbing trees, and having fun on the beach in Jamaica ended earlier than I wanted it to. Very abruptly I had to learn how to cope with the onslaught of technology, and a fast-paced culture built on fast food, fast fat, snack attacks, and heart attacks. I share all about my own food addictions and overweight before, during and after my pregnancy and my successful turnaround. And I did not stop at just losing the weight, but I built a championship physique. Follow me through my self-prescribed path from my overweight and pregnant state to my triumphant transformation as a body builder and overall winner of the first Ms. Natural California Contest and Ms Natural Fitness America.

Standing five feet one inch, I picked up my first pair of dumbbells after gaining over sixty pounds during my pregnancy. This was my first step on a journey of a thousand miles. My intentions were to trim the fat from the back of my arms and every where else. I desperately needed help all over. When you're barely over five feet tall, sixty pounds seems like a ton. Aerobically, I couldn't make it past two to three minutes. I felt like I was still carrying the baby on top of my abdomen instead of under it. During my attempt at a six-minute jog, my abdominal muscles were competing with my breasts. They were jumping ninety miles ahead of me. It felt like a big bowl of Jell-O. But before I tell you about the weight gain, the pregnancy, and my escape route, let me begin at the beginning.

My story began in the suburbs of Montego Bay, Jamaica where I lived the first ten years of my life. The land surrounding our house was scattered with fruit trees. My workout was climbing those trees. Dessert in Jamaica meant either climbing trees or chopping sugar cane. My childhood was a cross between that of a tomboy and a monkey. Swinging from branch to branch was the best back workout I've ever had. This might have been the foundation that helped me to win the "best back" trophy in body building in Okinawa, Japan, years later. Early investments do pay off. By the time I was in junior high school, I moved to New York City to join my Mom. My diet started changing on the plane ride to New York. For the first time in my life, I got a steak when I asked for it. For dessert I had the forbidden. It was very sweet, very rich, and very fattening. Can you imagine? The fat from the steak was satisfying. The "sugar high" from the dessert was intoxicating, and the ride in the sky was beyond cloud nine. I felt like I was in heaven, or at least on my way. After landing, we headed for Brooklyn, New York to see my brother who introduced us to American apple pie, sour cream pound cake, vanilla ice cream, and hot chocolate. Food I had never indulged in before was now in my possession. I exercised no mercy.

Island Girl Comes to Brooklyn

The sudden exposure to the New York winter awakened a giant appetite within me. A full stomach raised my body temperature and kept me warm and secure while television entertained me.

CONNECTION COMPLETE

Inevitably I developed the couch potato syndrome. My fear of facing the cold had me glued to the TV. Needless to say I became an instant addict in the junk food jungle. TV Commercials were the only cerebral exercise I got. In Jamaica, dinner took hours to prepare. Now, it was two minutes in the microwave. Wow! I was enjoying this. On Saturdays, my brothers and I went grocery shopping. The best part was buying all the junk we saw on television. Hiding under oversized sweaters and coats made me fail to realize that I'd gained over thirty five pounds in three months. I was in blissful denial failing to see that I had gained more than a quarter of my overall weight for my height. It dawned on me that the JFJ and my sedentary lifestyle had made me fat! With complete awe for America, I couldn't see that the average American diet was a piece of the junk food jungle, one meal after another. To me, junk food commercials were as enchanting as the magic of a good fairy tale. The JFJ appeals to all of our five senses. Just picture all the samples we can't walk past in the super markets. Yes, we indulge, but we all pay the piper sooner or later, either by being overweight or by developing deadly diseases. All the free samples that I was so grateful to devour were now a permanent fixture on my waistline. Not a pretty sight and summer was right around the corner. Should I run or hide? As the temperature and the humidity increased, I increased my fluid intake, which decreased my appetite. This was a blessing in disguise. With increased physical activity outdoors, I began to lose weight. By the next winter, my body did not react as intensely to hunger. I was determined not to regain the weight. My girl friend was on a diet because she was overweight. She was my deterrent from eating junk food. My sheltered, innocent, active, and healthy life in Jamaica was over. A four-hour plane ride had completely changed my future. For the first time, I knew I had to take responsibility for what I ate. Still it was just as hard for me to monitor what I ate as it was to resist temptations. Although food was new and appealing to me, I finally made the connection, that, being a couch potato and living in the junk food jungle could mean death in more ways than one. In Jamaica, I had eaten healthful foods in my ignorance. Now, I had to eat with a new awareness of healthful foods. I began my new healthy lifestyle by practicing the art of slow eating, but this was only temporary. By the time I moved away for college, I was short on cash and healthful foods. Once again, I was faced with the junk food jungle. After I finished college and began working as a registered nurse, I finally had money. My new problem was lack of time. Time to prepare a balanced meal was out of the question. I was caught up in the every day hustle and bustle of our contemporary stress. I had deadlines, schedules to adhere to, and overtime to cover for. I woke up to an alarm clock every morning at 5:30 with only enough time to shower, get dressed, and, ride the train to my 7:00 job. I went without breakfast most of the time. Sometimes we had donuts and coffee in the nurse's lounge. My diet was poor, hit or miss. I missed miserably most of the time. I became trapped in the spell, the lure, and the smell of the junk food jungle. There went my waistline. With youth on my side, I was still able to turn heads from time to time. After a few months as a nurse, I started dating a medical student. He earned his medical degree. We fell in love, married and soon I became pregnant.

The Pregnancy

This was another turning point in my life. I had unbelievable morning sickness. I literally could not keep anything down. Always starving, I was beginning to lose weight. However, in the third month of pregnancy after my morning sickness phase, I rapidly regained those lost pounds. I rediscovered food in a big way. My pregnancy was even more compelling than the cold weather. I was also feeling lonely and out of commission being alone in a new town. Food became my comfort, and my company. The urge to eat was as strong as a hungry lion with cubs. My days were filled with eating and sleeping. I panicked if I thought there wasn't enough food in the house. I discovered speed eating for the first time. I rationalized to myself that I had to eat for two, but two what? Three square meals and about four to six snack attacks was the order of my day. Even as a nurse, knowing the importance of a balanced diet during pregnancy, I found it impossible to adhere to. My desire to eat all the time was so strong that I couldn't control myself. To be honest I didn't want to. I wanted to sit my butt down, and eat all that I

CONNECTION COMPLETE

desired and I did. Exercise was boring and demanding, I avoided that. Sleep was easier. Every two-three hours I felt like a great dane although I would prefer to have felt like a grand dame. I felt like I had only two choices, eat, or die. Well what would you do? Exactly, that's what I did too. I lived in fear of hunger. On trips that were over an hour long, I would take lots of food in the car to placate my anxiety. Once, I was caught in the Christmas rush in Manhattan, stranded without food in the middle of rush-hour traffic. That experience stirred up a lot of anxiety in me towards food. I felt like my life was on the line. I would have done anything for food. I just wanted to eat. Looking back on my experience as a nursing supervisor in a chemical dependency hospital, I can safely compare my passion for food to that of a drug addict going through withdrawal symptoms. It was my only cure for the pain. My pregnancy went well and my weight gain was in generous portions for my height. I must confess, I never, thought I could get so big, just like I never realized that I could eat the whole thing...what ever that happened to be. Albeit, pregnancy does one good thing, it increases the metabolic rate of the body, allowing it to burn more calories even without exercise. Unfortunately, pregnancy does not change our ability to inflate fat cells. So when we go on an **all-you-can-eat diet**, the reality can be devastating to our figure, our health, and the way we feel about our selves. Early in my ninth month of pregnancy I had already gained fifty six pounds! This is about half of my ideal weight for my height. I looked in the mirror only to see a woman I did not recognize. I asked myself, "Who is this person?" I had difficulty getting dressed, wanting to look and feel attractive but instead feeling like the circus fat lady. It was humbling and a crush to my pride. I felt robbed of my femininity and my sex appeal. I didn't feel attractive, and I didn't think my husband found me attractive any longer. I can remember once I got all dressed up in a purple outfit, pretending that I was sexier than ever. Out of the blue, my husband said to me, "That outfit is supposed to be sexy?" It was as if he had said, "You're not sexy. You're pregnant." I just smiled and thought to myself, I still want to feel like an attractive woman though. He reacted to my being pregnant as though I had become brain dead, unappealing and was now just a pregnant body.

While he struggled with his ambivalence toward me, I felt like a prisoner behind my fat and pregnant belly. I could see how aesthetically unattractive he found the anatomical changes of pregnancy on a woman. I lost interest in taking pictures while I was fat and pregnant. I even felt somewhat ashamed of my appearance. I thought about all the women I'd heard say that their husbands were uninterested in them after the baby because they were fat. Being the fighter that I am, I developed an intense desire to take charge of my body once I delivered my baby. My level of insecurity about my appearance was at a record high. Never again, I thought. Finally, the day came on September 22, 1983 at 9:00 p.m. when my six pound, nine ounce, son, Eric arrived into my world, oh what a blessing he was, I thought. Now I have a special reason to live a healthy lifestyle.

Recovering From Pregnancy and Delivery

On September 23, I looked eight months pregnant instead of nine. My new long-term goal was to lose the weight permanently within a year. That was the day of my mantra. **I'm into health for the long haul.** Even while still in the hospital, I started doing abdominal crunches. I linked so much pain to my body image that I had to take action right away to change things. I refused to grow fat gracefully. I also started breast-feeding, a big plus for Eric and for me. The day I came home, as I went through my closet I couldn't find any thing to fit me. Frankly, my three days of abdominal flexing was as significant as the bite of a flea on the hide of a dinosaur. My favorite jeans could barely come up above my knees. After waiting all those months to fit into my old wardrobe I was disappointed, and angry, realizing that I had a nightmare of a job ahead of me. I could feel the biggest lump in my throat as I left the hospital to face my new life. Getting back to normal physically and raising my son was paramount. With a little help from Mother Nature, breast-feeding proved to be a wise decision.

Breast Feeding and my Weight Loss

Having experienced the benefits of weight loss while breast-feeding, I am now quite an advocate of breast milk for babies. Mother Nature made it a natural and healthy bonding for mother and child. Do you remember the acquired fat during your early teens? That's the reserve fuel that Mother Nature gave us women to feed our babies. This is the fat that becomes available for nursing babies. It ensures survival of the species. This fat is accumulated around the hips and buttocks and is very difficult to lose during weight loss attempts. The pregnant body goes through magic in the last trimester of pregnancy. The milk-producing hormone called prolactin becomes more abundant. This increased hormone level allows such difficult fat cells to be accessible for milk production. This milk production burns approximately 800 extra calories. Nursing was instrumental in burning unwanted body fat more rapidly from problem areas.

Japan: A New Awakening

My husband and I were scheduled to move to Atsugi, Japan for three years following orders from the U.S. Navy. I felt that my pregnancy and my child's birth were big adjustments in our young marriage. However, our move to Japan made the stresses of pregnancy and childbirth seem minute. This was stressful news for me to digest. The junk food jungle was tempting me at every turn again. I was curious about Japanese cuisine and I was home sick for some American as well as Jamaican foods. Now I had three cultures clashing within my mind and my taste buds. Do I dare to enter the jungle out of boredom, nostalgia or curiosity? What if I got lost there? Maybe I needed to deal with my feelings and stress level appropriately. I sought professional help. I knew that moving is on the top of the stress list, but I also knew that the junk food jungle was not the place to resolve stress. After settling in Japan I pursued my goal to get in the best physical condition that I possibly could, before returning to the US. Our first home was a military hut on the naval base. I established an exercise schedule at home and

Marcia Sheridan, R.N.

a month later, I was able to do two to three twenty minute sessions of aerobics. I was already feeling better than I had before my pregnancy. Exercising was great for venting stress, and passing the time. My promise to my son and to myself to achieve health and fitness kept me moving. Soon I was almost an aerobics expert having increased my time and stamina to two hours. Desire was now propelling me. It was no longer my husband's reaction. Secretly he was surprised and pleased with my progress after months of hard work. I started taking walks with Eric in order to familiarize myself with the base. On one of my walks, I noticed an enormous air plane hangar that said "gymnasium" on the front. This really got my attention. It was something else to add to my 'to-do list'—go to the gym! But instead, I started running about five miles three times a week. I wanted to walk into this gym looking great, not looking like I had just had a baby. As a nurse, I had seen lots of women who had gotten fatter and fatter after each baby. They never seemed to get back to normal. I can remember as a nursing student that two out of three of my classmates were continually on, and off diets. They would say to me, "I used to be exactly your size, until I had kids. You better enjoy your figure now. After you have babies you'll never look petite again." The one smart thing I did was not to believe that thought of never. My mom told me to never let other people decide for me what I could and can never do. I promised myself that I would not lose myself to obesity, and that I would not become Marcia the Fat Mamma. Feeling insecure about my looks was a situation not to be revisited ever again. I made a decision to find the inner source of strength that would see me through the long haul of health and fitness. Finally I boldly walked into the gym one afternoon to ride the stationary bike. An active duty officer saw me and said, "You look great. Are you an aerobics instructor?" I told her I was there to enroll in an aerobics class. She replied, "We are greatly in need of an instructor and you look like one. Would you like to teach a class?" Flattered and enthusiastic, I said "yes" without hesitation. You never know when you spontaneously throw a pebble in the ocean how far the circles will take you. In my case it will take me through my entire life in good health. The next week, I went to my first class of seven students. This was the first time I had ever been in an aerobics class. The first thirty minutes was quite long. I was surprised to see that these people could barely keep up with me. Albeit, we made it through the hour, I was expecting the class to be more advanced than I was. I had put my best foot forward, and surprised myself. I started two other classes, one for the advanced and one for beginners. This worked well for six months. Meanwhile, I developed the stamina of a racehorse. A year went by, and my goal was more than realized. What's next? My legs caught the attention of the Officers Wives Club. I was invited to model short kimonos as their featured attraction at the Officers Club. The most memorable moment for me was my invitation to be the first American to demonstrate aerobics to the Japanese in the Atsugi-Yokohama area. This was in the eighties when aerobics were first coming into vogue. They all brought their cameras and asked politely to take photos of me. The president of the group brought me gifts of recipe books, Japanese food, and money. I felt special and appreciated that day. This experience was a strong encouragement for me to keep improving my physique. I began to dream of getting into a competitive sport, only I wasn't sure what it should be. I continued to jog five miles and ride my bike daily. Female body builders inspired me. I wanted that look. Finally my decision was made. Bodybuilding it would be. I even had visions of competing some day. After a few weeks in the gym, I broke the ice by teaching a class in female bodybuilding. I chose bodybuilding because I wanted to get stronger. My decision was also based on convenience, access to a gym, and curiosity about women's potential in muscle building. I wanted to see how fast, and how far I could take my body in developing muscularity. As soon as I made the decision, I was overwhelmed with energy and enthusiasm. Making the right decisions is the first and best way to flex one's muscles. I became passionate and focused on my goal. My daily routine was to ride my bike with my son. Those were some of the most memorable moments for me. What better way to be with my baby? I was getting fit, having fun, and being free with my child. Each lap was about forty five minutes around the perimeter of the base with three challenging, steep hills. The freedom I felt riding made the time fly like the wind, effortlessly. While others stressfully pushed their bikes over the hills, I changed gears, and slowly cranked my way over for that million-dollar thrill. Eric was a good sport. He enjoyed every minute with me. My bodybuilding routine was to work legs and shoulders the first day, chest and triceps the second day, back and biceps the third day, and abdominal muscles, forearms, and calves every day. I rested on the fourth day and on Sundays when I go to church with my family. I repeated the same routine all over again on Monday. This allowed me to work each body part twice per week. By rotating work on each body part, and allowing two days of rest for each part, I was able to work harder and longer. When I first started, I could barely last for six minutes, but I found out that when I am most stressed I benefit the most from my workouts. Exercise was the best therapy for my stress. It harmonized my physical energy with my spiritual energy perfectly. On this rotation program, I developed significant size in nine months to a year. I trimmed off my excess fat nicely, and was quite toned. I could see my body looking like a pro. I had visions of a new Marcia. For the first time, I saw a different woman when I looked in the mirror. I often had tears of joy and a sense of accomplishment. Looking in the mirror before a workout would motivate me to chisel an ounce of fat from various places. As a physique sculptor, I used the mirror as my guide instead of the scale. I could see that my weight gain was muscles and my weight loss was fat. My compulsion to jump on the scale was lost. I learned the mirror was really a more accurate scale; it reflected the true picture of what I looked like. After regular aerobics and a straight year of hard labor in the gym, my makeover emerged. I saw an almost fat-free body, symmetrical, strong, athletic, and pleasing to my eyes. This experience convinced me that people have an innate ability to do the impossible. During my attempt to be a sculptor like Michelangelo, I fought through a myriad of physical and emotional barriers. There were days when my body would respond to the weather. I must tell you staying on the course was like being on a battleground. I got attacked from all angles. It was only the strength of my spirit that kept me fighting to reach my goal. On a cloudy rainy day, or on certain days in the month, I struggled with winter depression (called seasonal affective disorder) feelings of staying in bed, skipping my workout, and cheating on my diet. To be frank, sometimes I did just that. However, my burning desire to stay healthy for the long haul kept me going. My winning attitude and spiritual connection helped me to dismiss negative phases when they come. I never allowed myself to be deterred from my goals and purpose for long. Sometimes I went back mentally to when I was a nursing student. I remembered the inner strength and potential I had to reach into myself for energy and drive. I always found my "psychophysical" self, my sense of personal power. My athletic skills, mental training, spiritual awareness, and social and family life were orchestrated to produce a satisfied and balanced woman being.

The Connection Payoff

After a few months of psychophysical (mind/body) type workouts, I began to feel that I could do the impossible. I knew the surge of power I discovered inside of me could erase my doubts and negative emotions and release the drive and perseverance I needed to be on purpose. I was beginning to enjoy the feeling of being wholesome. Our time was ending in Japan, and I was longing to go home. I had dreams of competing more and more every day. I could see myself clearly, as I wanted to be, believing that I could make it happen. This journey is long and lonely but winners don't quit. Finally, at the end of three long years, my family and I moved back to Southern California, a most welcomed relief—a haven for bodybuilding. A few months later, I joined Holiday Spa, a real gym with modern equipment. I felt like a kid in a candy store playing with all the weights. My enthusiasm was overwhelming. I sentenced myself to three months of hard labor (train like a pro). At this time I took a full time job as a nursing supervisor at Care Unit Hospital. I trained every day after work and on Saturdays for four hours. I became friends with a marine power lifter, Jim, who later became my training partner. We had some dynamite workouts together. We just seemed to give each other the last ounce of strength we needed to get that extra repetition. My first contest was the biggest thrill I've ever experienced. The producer of Hercules USA bodybuilding contest invited me to enter. His first comment was

Marcia Sheridan, R.N.

"Where have you been? You look great. I can't think of anyone looking better than you." To meet someone with so much faith in me gave me the confidence to finally go for it. I had three long weeks of hard training. I was determined to be completely defined and fat free for this contest. I wanted a first place trophy for Eric. It's amazing how much one can transform in three weeks when driven. Dreams and goals can really break down our crippling belief system, and move mountains as soon as we take action. On the day of the contest, I was mentally, physically and spiritually ready. I focused on impressing the judges on my first walk out on stage. I could feel my heart pounding against my chest. When the audience screamed, I wanted to jump out of my skin with excitement. Luckily, this worked in my favor. The judges enjoyed my energy and excitement in addition to what they called my outstanding physique. I won the first place and the overall trophy (my first). I was proud of the results of my accomplishments. I entered another contest a week later. There was a little more competition for me at this contest, but I walked away with the first place and overall trophy, again. Back stage, I was pulled aside by some admiring fans. Yes! I had a fan club. They suggested I enter the Orange County Muscle Classic contest only three weeks away. Once again, too naive about the sport to question anything, I thought, "Well, three more weeks won't kill me." However, it was quite a drain on my body having to diet and work out continuously for over seven weeks, which is something I will never do again. The Orange County Muscle Classic is a wonderful title to have. It is the largest show of its type in America, staged yearly at Disneyland. Most of the top Ms. Olympia contestants received their first big break here. National exposure on television, and in several magazines, comes with this title. Naturally, I wanted the title and the exposure. To ensure winning, I started running five miles per day up hill with wrist weights. Running helped to keep my metabolism high and my body fat burning. It helped me to maintain my muscle tone and definition. I also went on a split routine workout by training my upper body in the mornings, and working my lower body at night. I took a nap after lunch, took care of Eric until after dinner, and then went to the gym again. Adhering to this routine for three more weeks was a nightmare. But the

CONNECTION COMPLETE

toughest challenge was to stay on my diet in spite of the television temptations and the occasional scent of junk food. Once I did break down and ate some cookies. I really felt like having the entire bag of cookies. To stop myself, I decided to go riding with Eric. My parental responsibility came first. This was actually rather refreshing since we had short talks along the way just like we did in Japan. Finally, the Rancho Santa Margarita Hill in Mission Viejo was in front of me. It was steep and seemed at least a mile long. I realized Eric weighed more than thirty pounds and my bike was old. Riding over the hill was doubtful but the challenge was too tempting. I had to face that hill. At the bottom of the hill I was passed by a group of cyclists who turned around and looked at me with pity, as if they thought I was a crazy housewife who should at best push the bike over the hill. So I turned up the speed of my bike and went at it with full force. I thought of Emily Dickinson "hope is the thing with feathers that perches in the soul", I was hoping to fly over the hill on my bike. Occasionally, they glanced, out of curiosity. I kept cranking thinking of the past in Japan and my future in the contest. My son kept saying, "Go, Mom, Go!" I could feel my heart beating at what must have been 200 beats per minute. Since my heart rate had never been that high before, I kept praying that I wouldn't have a heart attack. The closer I got to the top, the farther it seemed. The cyclists were still in sight and they could see that I had made it in spite of my old bike and carrying Eric's thirty extra pounds. I have never felt such inner and outer power in my life. The cyclists were all men over six feet tall. They rode like pros, dressed like pros, and looked like pros. When they got to the end of the trail they turned around to face me on their way back. I wore a big smile of triumph, while they tried to hide their astonishment by hanging their heads down, avoiding eye contact with me. This experience reminded me of my last contest when I could see Mike, a workout acquaintance from my gym, in the audience as I won the Overall Trophy. However, while we worked out together the next week, he never even mentioned to me that he was there until I asked him about it. I then realized that some people resent the success of others. The sense of victory and the confirmation I felt with my experience with the cyclists was just too much. I had to stop and jump up and down, screaming to my son, "Eric, I did it! I did it! I really did it!" "Mom, I knew you would," he said. I was the little woman being who had the courage to tackle the mountain on her old bike. At that moment I pictured myself winning the Orange County Muscle Classic. My inner source told me I was invincible. And I believed it. I told everyone I knew about my experience on the Santa Margarita Hill. This was a little bit of madness that kept me going. Every time I pictured this episode and remembered the euphoria, my workouts got easier, I even enjoyed them. But even more, even today I draw energy and inspiration from that one action I took at that one short magnificent moment in time. A time that is forever etched in my heart because it represents a piece a strength lifted out of the depths of my soul. I discovered this dept through a physical action but today I know how to connect with that source just by my intention. This is a key that I use in all aspects of my life, I can't tell you what a profound experience it was for me. It has taught me, to always associate past victories with anticipated ones. Such memories give us the magic to move forward. So I promised my son the first place trophy. I made another connection, how to have faith before I take actions. Having my son watch me win a big trophy for him was for sure. I wanted to be a role model for Eric just as much as all of his sports idols. So what if I'm a woman. It's the dawning of a new millenium all things are possible when we believe. Fathers are not always the athletes in the family or the inspiration for their sons' sports careers. This gift was to come from mother to son. I feel privileged to be the inspiration for my child. He gave me the inner strength to enter this contest with confidence. On May 5, 1987, the moment of truth arrived. I was the last contestant to weigh in at the prejudging. I kept to myself as usual until just before going on stage and surprising every one. I just kept smiling through my individual routine. I felt such a relief at the end that a loud scream came out of my mouth, shocking the judges, as well as myself. They all smiled. Back-stage, the coordinator of the show said to me, "That's good; you showed your feelings. The judges like that". I left very satisfied with my performance. We drove back to Disneyland at 5:00 p.m. Like a true athlete I visualized the evening; with me in a gold bikini, with oil all over my body, standing in front of six thousand people posing like the champ. My enthusiasm was flowing, I could feel the excitement. I could hear the roar of the crowd. I could see myself walking away with the first place and the overall trophies. I realized the judges were doing a good job in picking the best person. Something inside of me clicked. I knew that I would break a record and become the first lightweight female to win the coveted overall title for the Ms. Orange County Contest at Disney Land. The big moment came when I heard my name and number. I ran on stage, waited for my music, and then went into a trance as I performed my posing routine. This is when we flex our muscles in a sort of dance routine for the audience's entertainment and for the judges to see us a second time before they announce the winner. There was a silence, even the wind held it's breath, but I did not panic. I continued on with the moonwalk, completed my routine, blew the audience a kiss, and vanished. Minutes later we were back on stage for the pose down and trophy presentation. This went very fast. I remember hearing, "And the winner of the light-weight class is number 124, Marcia Sheridan." As I left the stage in excitement, I was told to stay for the overall pose down with the middle-weight and heavy-weight women. This was like a circus. These women were huge next to me. Would my slingshot work this time? We'll see. Before I could get used to my first place trophy, I was back on stage fighting for a seven foot trophy. The judges made me work for this one. They kept comparing us against each other, then we had a chance to breathe. The wait was similar to the Miss America beauty contest. Finally, Mary Roberts, former Ms. Olympia contestant, said, "Would you please give the Overall Trophy to contestant number 124, Marcia Sheridan." I jumped, I screamed, and I danced. I blew kisses to the audience. I posed for the magazine photographers, and then went crazy back stage. Here I was the mother of a four and a half-year-old son winning an overall title against girls in their teens. The best part was that they had no idea I was not one of them. I became successful only because I believed deeply that I could.

Marcia Sheridan, R.N.

The Greatest Challenge

Winning the Ms. Orange County title was great. It qualified me to enter the women's nationals, the Ms. Natural America Fitness (bodybuilding) contest. I also got a surprise call from friends telling me that my picture was in Flex magazine, a nice treat for a novice. With this title, I wanted to go on to the nationals. I felt I could do no wrong. Nationals were five months away. This was the title that would turn me into a professional body builder, one of Joe Weider's girls. Again I had no plans to go this far. Health and fitness alone would be my wildest dream come true. I had to see how far I could go while I was still having fun. I made plans to take two months to rest my body before I resumed training for the nationals. I took six weeks off, moved to Pasadena from Orange County, and joined a new gym. It was June 1987 when I went back into heavy training. I went in early one morning to work my back and arms. My enthusiasm had me working hard and heavy right from the beginning. I seemed to have forgotten that I was ever off training. On my last set of dead lifts for the lower back, I decided to do one extra repetition—one that I'm still paying for today. On the recovery phase, my back snapped. I felt pain, and I dropped the weights. I went home, took a muscle relaxant and went to bed. Bright and early the next morning, I jumped on my stationary bike to warm up, pretending my back was just fine. After about ten seconds, I could feel real pain creeping up from my tailbone to my lower back. I realized that I had just worsened my condition by ignoring it. I could be seriously injured. This meant going back to bed in more pain than I had the day before. This was a lesson in patience, and dealing with an injury that I'll never forget. I hated not being able to work out. Every day counts, especially when there were only three months to build muscles and then break them down for definition before a major contest. My condition progressively got worse over the next week, contrary to my expectations. At this point I was getting through the first stage of the grieving process called denial. Reality then started to set in. I was accepting the strong possibility that I would have to skip the contest. Severe back spasms led to severe pain that kept me off my feet. I had difficulty climbing stairs, walking in high-heeled shoes, standing for long periods, sitting, and lying flat on my back. Every position caused painful muscle spasms. My condition worsened to the point where I became bedridden. My husband, a physician, prescribed muscle relaxants and anti-inflammatory medications for me. He suggested two weeks of bed rest, with my leg elevated to keep pressure off the lower back. These two weeks turned into six months of agony. I tried traction in bed. I went to a chiropractor for treatments. I went to an orthopedic surgeon who prescribed more drugs. I spent six months taking pain medications, which did not kill the pain but instead kept me drowsy and lethargic. Lying on my back throughout the fall and winter months gave me time to question what happened to me, why it happened, and how I was going to recover. Where do I go from here? I was feeling lonely, helpless and depressed. I felt disconnected from life when I badly needed a connection. Knowing that negative feelings would destroy me, I went back in time to a period in my life when I felt invincible. I watched videotapes of my contests, which stirred up old memories and feelings. I had forgotten about the good feelings I had about myself. I held onto the tapes and the feelings for renewal in my spirit. I was about to rebuild my mental and spiritual muscles, and heal myself. I prayed a lot. I could not spend any more of my life lying on my back in pain. I fantasized about being able to compete again. Positive thoughts became a powerful force in my life. And then I remembered the moment, the Santa Marguirita Hill that I once climbed on an old bike. I started to perceive and to believe that I could once again achieve my dreams. I wasn't able to go to church for a long while so I watched The Hour of Power with Robert Schuller on Sundays which was a blessing and an inspiration to my spirit. I was feeding my mind and working out mentally. I used this time to strengthen my inner and outer muscles and to connect to my inner source of creation. Spring brought hope along with new life. Birds were singing at my window, and my spirit quickened with energy. I felt like I did back in Jamaica, begging to come alive and whole again. Sunny days, singing birds, blue skies, and green grass got me hopping around outside. It was warm enough for the pool. I started swimming an hour a day followed by doing stretching and calisthenics. The first experience was incredible.

My back felt loose. In fact my whole body became loose and relaxed. I finally had my first good night's sleep after six months of emotional and physical agony. I felt as if I was being awakened from a long nightmare. I knew the road to recovery would be long. But with my renewed spirit I was completely ready to be self-empowered. An unexplainable feeling came over me. I felt like a miracle was about to unfold in my life. I was able to look at my injury from a different perspective. It became an opportunity to overcome. I knew that if I were able to overcome this setback, I would be a lot stronger both physically and spiritually. I remember clearly the incredible realization that I could command of my life with the help of divine guidance. This was the source of my will to take charge. I could turn my scars into stars, according to Schuller. I believed him. I stopped expecting help from outside. I was determined to heal myself by completely connecting to my inner source of strength. I relied on my faith and my self-determination to see me through this. But that was not enough to keep me out of the junk food jungle. I was still bored and frustrated. I was visiting the jungle occasionally to enjoy some of my old friends, like cookies, ice cream, and chocolate. Not to worry; I was still in for the long haul so I bounce back better than ever. Just the acorn of faith I needed came ringing through my telephone. Mike Glass, the producer of the Orange county Muscle Classic called. He said, "Marcia, I was just looking at the video of you on my last show and you are the most electrifying performer that I've ever seen. You seem like you were really having a great time at my last show. We need someone like you to help promote this new show I'm doing. Would you be able to guest pose? It's only about two months away, but I hear you always look great." I felt honored. I knew that I was still in great shape after six months of bed rest. I told him nothing of my injury, I just accepted the honor with gratitude. It was a great opportunity to get back on stage without the stresses of competition. My first step was to work out a schedule for the month including my music and my routine. Then I began to visualize in my mind precisely the way I wanted to look, feel, and perform on stage. I stood in front of a full-length mirror in my bikini and critiqued my body. My bed rest cost me about eight pounds of muscles, and I had gained a few pounds of fat. I was quite lean, however. I needed to build five pounds of muscle to tone up. The plan was to also adhere to a low fat, high carbohydrate, moderate protein diet. As it turned out, I could last for only two hours in the mornings. I also needed a two-hour rest. In the evenings, I would swim and stretch. With my strong determination to make a comeback, I got physical therapy and massage therapy twice every week, all the while enduring great pain with a smile. Before I knew it, I was standing in the dark and being introduced. Then suddenly, I was hit with the spotlight, the music, and the audience. My body began to move automatically, my heart was in it, and I gave it all I had. There were tears of joy, a dance of freedom, a fit body and a spirit that did not quit. I showered the audience with love, enthusiasm, and passion. In return, they expressed much appreciation. They screamed in enjoyment. The six months of agony flashed through my mind—it seemed like minutes. At that moment, I felt larger than life. I was proud of my decision and my will to follow through. It was the best trophy I could win, my own self-confidence.

My second chance to be a part of life? The California Natural a drug-free contest, what a great idea. I decided, I must have this title. This was the first NPC Natural California Contest (drug free contest). I decided to enter to make a moral statement against drugs. I had seven weeks of hard work ahead of me for this contest. It was now easier for me to go into a contest knowing that I was back in shape and in circulation. I was almost my old self again. I reflected on my childhood in Jamaica climbing trees, my pregnancy, gaining sixty pounds, and my first contest. I realized that I had been very blessed and I thanked God for giving me a second chance. My seven weeks of hard labor paid off. I won the first place and the overall title for the first Ms. Natural California, a tremendous milestone for me. A few weeks later, I had a write up in Natural Physique magazine with a nice full-body color picture. A month later, I entered the Natural Nationals for the Miss Natural All American. This was also a drug-tested contest held only in Redondo Beach California every year. I won my first place title for Ms. Natural America, 1988, a dream come true. I drove home from Redondo Beach with my trophy feeling that I had gone as far as I could go in

Marcia Sheridan, R.N.

drug-free bodybuilding. I could become one of Joe Weider's body building babes or I could move on as my own person. Taking drugs was out of the question, I was satisfied with my achievements. I made guest appearances on other shows, such as the Laguna Beach Muscle Classic for Ken Norton (once heavy weight champion of the world). In fact we even discussed the possibility of me training with him before he opened his Golds Gym in El Toro California. However after I guessed posed for Ken Norton's Show in Laguna Beach California my spirit was calling me into a different direction. I decided to retire from competition, and start nursing again. I had learned the lessons that I was meant to learn through the physical path. It was time to move on, to make contributions from what I had learned. I took with me my knowledge, a fit and healthy body, great discipline, and a burning passion for mindful, healthful living. I refuse to compete anymore, not even in my Toast Masters speeches. I watch other people win; it's more fun. As a registered nurse, mother, wife, and athlete, I'm aspiring to be a beacon of light to help women escape the stress, destruction and disease of the junk food jungle. I am now an active speaker for the American Cancer Society and the American Heart Association to help educate and empower women to move into the new millenium with a new mantra. One that will help them to completely connect to their authentic purpose on this planet. I now conduct group seminars, and one on one consultations. I will be teaching health and fitness in the colleges soon. I'm active as a motivational professional speaker in health and fitness, stress management, and personal empowerment for corporations, associations, and women's groups. I have shared with you my medical knowledge as a registered nurse, my experience as an over-weight mother, my athletic knowledge as Miss Fitness America, my spiritual wisdom and awakening, and most of all my passion to persuade, to inform, and to inspire. Are you ready ladies? Let us all unite and escape the junk food jungle, understand and survive contemporary stress, reunite with our spiritual source of creation, live consciously, stick to health and fitness for the long haul, actualize our heart's desire as a collective spiritual force for the long haul. If you now feel like you have the gift of knowledge and enlightenment please allow others to light their candle from it,

CONNECTION COMPLETE

keep it circulating. Donate your copy to a library or give it as a gift to friends and the power of the knowledge will be yours forever. What ever we desire deeply we should first give away. It will come back in abundance. In this way we can expedite our global spiritual growth and development, fulfill our authentic heart's desire and completely connect to collective divine purpose. Although we may never meet in person, we are now united as one love in the spirit.

Marcia Sheridan, R.N.

TO ARRANGE A WORKSHOP, LECTURE OR SPEAKING ENGAGEMENT:

E-mail: Msheridan@Ameritech.Net
or contact the Publisher at:
Sterlinghouse Publisher
440 Friday Road, Pittsburgh, PA 15209
1-888-542-BOOK
sterlingho@aol.com

CONNECTION COMPLETE

GLOSSARY

Abdomen \ ab-do-men: the portion of the body below the thorax

Aerobics \ er-ro-bik: in the presence of oxygen, a system of exercise that increases the respirations, and heart rate.

Albumin \ al'bu-min: a simple protein found in most animal, and vegetable tissues.

Angioplasty \ an'jeo- plas-te: plastic repair of blood vessels or lymphatic channels.

Atherosclerosis \ ath' er- o- skle-ro-sis: a form of arteriosclerosis, cholesterol/fatty materials formed within large and medium-sized arteries.

Bicepts \ bi-seps: a muscle in the upper arm with two heads, it flexes, and extends the forearm.

BMR \ Basal Metabolic Rate: a measurement of the expenditure of energy by measuring the rate of oxygen intake, and expenditure.

Buttocks\ (but-ok): the two fleshy prominences formed by the gluteal muscles on the end of the lower back.

Coma \ ko-mah: a state of unconsciousness from which there is no arousal even with powerful stimuli.

CBC \ complete blood count: blood cell count.

Derriere \ der-e-er: buttocks, or see buttocks above.

CONNECTION COMPLETE

Diastasis Recti Abdominis \ di-as'tah-sis reck' tye ab-do-i-nis: separation in the median line of the two rectus abdominus muscles in the abdomen.

Diverticulitis \ dye-ver.tick' yoo.lye-tis: inflamation in the colon, (within the diverticula).

Episiotomy \ e-piz-' ee. ot'uh.mee: medical incision of the vulva (within the vaginal area) during child birth, to avoid undue laceretion.

Exacerbation \ eg.zas'ur.bay'shun: to irritate, an increase in the manifestations or severity of a disease or symptom.

Fatal \ fay-tul: deadly disasterous.

Fetal \ fee'tul: pertaining to a fetus.

Fetus \ fe'tus: the developing young in the uterus.

Hemorhage \ hem'uh. Ridj: an escape of blood from the vessels.

Girth \ gerth: the measurement around the waist.

Glycemia \ gli-se-mia: the presence of glucose in the blood.

Herniation \ hur-nee-a-tion: the abnormal protrusion of a part through the containing wall of its cavity.

Hiatal Hernia \ hia.tal her'-ne-ah: the protrusion of of a portion of the stomach through the esophageal hiatus of the stomach.

Insoluble \ in-sol-u-b'l: not susceptable of being disolved.

Insulin \ in'su-lin: a protein hormone that regulates, carbohydrate, protein, lipids, and amino acid (protein) metabolism.

Krebs Cycle \ krebz, tricarboxylic acid cycle \ tri'car-bok-sil'ik: the cyclic metabolic mechanism by which the carbon chains of sugars, fatty acids, and amino acid are metabolized to yield carbon dioxide water, and high energy-energy phosphate bonds. Called also citric acid cycle.

Nasogastric tube \ na-zo-gas'trik: a tube that funnels the food through the nose down into the stomach.

Nephron \ nef"ron: the structural, and functional unit of the kidneys that form urine.

Osteoporosis \ os'te-o-po-ro-sis: abnormal thinning of bones.

Pelvic \ pel'vik: hip bone, comprising of the elium, ischium, and pelvis.

Perineum \ per-I-ne-um: the pelvic floor, and associated structure occupying the pelvic outlet.

Peristalsis \ per'I-stal'sis: movement by which the intestines propel its content.

Prolapse \ pro'laps: falling down, downward displacement of a body part.

Prone \ pron: lying face down.

Quadriceps \ kwod-ri-seps: the four head of muscles in the anterior upper thigh.

Rectum \ rek' tum: the end of the anal canal, anus, distal portion of the large intestine.

Repetition \ repe-ti-tion: the act of repeating.

CONNECTION COMPLETE

Shock \ shok: disruption of the circulation which can upset all body functions, and or lead to death.

Soluble \ sol-u-b'l: susceptible to being dissolved.

Squats \ skwat: the lowering of body (posture) to the ground by bending knees over toes during exercise, with or without weights on shoulders.

Supine \ su-pin: lying on the back, or lying face down.

Syndrome \ sin-drom: a combination of symptoms.

Thrombolytic \ throm-bo-lit-ik: dessolving or splitting up a solid mass formed in the heart or blood vessels.

Marcia Sheridan, R.N.

CONNECTION COMPLETE